Priska Vonbach

**Drug-Drug Interactions in the Hospital**

Priska Vonbach

# Drug-Drug Interactions in the Hospital

Südwestdeutscher Verlag für Hochschulschriften

**Impressum/Imprint (nur für Deutschland/ only for Germany)**
Bibliografische Information der Deutschen Nationalbibliothek: Die Deutsche Nationalbibliothek verzeichnet diese Publikation in der Deutschen Nationalbibliografie; detaillierte bibliografische Daten sind im Internet über http://dnb.d-nb.de abrufbar.
Alle in diesem Buch genannten Marken und Produktnamen unterliegen warenzeichen-, markenoder patentrechtlichem Schutz bzw. sind Warenzeichen oder eingetragene Warenzeichen der jeweiligen Inhaber. Die Wiedergabe von Marken, Produktnamen, Gebrauchsnamen, Handelsnamen, Warenbezeichnungen u.s.w. in diesem Werk berechtigt auch ohne besondere Kennzeichnung nicht zu der Annahme, dass solche Namen im Sinne der Warenzeichen- und Markenschutzgesetzgebung als frei zu betrachten wären und daher von jedermann benutzt werden dürften.

Verlag: Südwestdeutscher Verlag für Hochschulschriften Aktiengesellschaft & Co. KG
Dudweiler Landstr. 99, 66123 Saarbrücken, Deutschland
Telefon +49 681 37 20 271-1, Telefax +49 681 37 20 271-0, Email: info@svh-verlag.de
Zugl.: Basel, University of Basel, Dissertation, 2007

Herstellung in Deutschland:
Schaltungsdienst Lange o.H.G., Berlin
Books on Demand GmbH, Norderstedt
Reha GmbH, Saarbrücken
Amazon Distribution GmbH, Leipzig
ISBN: 978-3-8381-0462-1

**Imprint (only for USA, GB)**
Bibliographic information published by the Deutsche Nationalbibliothek: The Deutsche Nationalbibliothek lists this publication in the Deutsche Nationalbibliografie; detailed bibliographic data are available in the Internet at http://dnb.d-nb.de.
Any brand names and product names mentioned in this book are subject to trademark, brand or patent protection and are trademarks or registered trademarks of their respective holders. The use of brand names, product names, common names, trade names, product descriptions etc. even without a particular marking in this works is in no way to be construed to mean that such names may be regarded as unrestricted in respect of trademark and brand protection legislation and could thus be used by anyone.

Publisher:
Südwestdeutscher Verlag für Hochschulschriften Aktiengesellschaft & Co. KG
Dudweiler Landstr. 99, 66123 Saarbrücken, Germany
Phone +49 681 37 20 271-1, Fax +49 681 37 20 271-0, Email: info@svh-verlag.de

Copyright © 2009 by the author and Südwestdeutscher Verlag für Hochschulschriften Aktiengesellschaft & Co. KG and licensors
All rights reserved. Saarbrücken 2009

Printed in the U.S.A.
Printed in the U.K. by (see last page)
**ISBN: 978-3-8381-0462-1**

Dedicated to my parents and to Lukas

## Acknowledgements

I would like to express my sincerest thanks to Prof. Dr. Dr. Stephan Krähenbühl (Clinical Pharmacology & Toxicology, University Hospital Basel), Prof. Dr. Jürg H. Beer (Department of Medicine, Cantonal Hospital of Baden) and Dr. André Dubied (Hospital Pharmacy, Cantonal Hospital of Baden) for the opportunity of working on this fascinating project in the field of clinical pharmacy. I greatly appreciate their assistance with organizing the studies, analyzing the results and writing the publications. They supported me with important suggestions, but allowed me the freedom to carry out the studies independently, without losing focus on the objective.

Furthermore, I would like to thank Prof. Dr. Jürgen Drewe (Clinical Pharmacology & Toxicology, University Hospital Basel) for his recommendation letter to the Faculty of Natural Science and Prof. Dr. M. Hamburger (Pharmaceutical Biology, Department of Pharmaceutical Sciences, University of Basel) for heading my doctor examination.

My thanks go also to Prof. Dr. P.E. Ballmer (Department of Medicine, Cantonal Hospital of Winterthur) for his cooperativeness and for the inspiring discussions.

I wish to address my thanks to PD Dr. Christoph R. Meier (Basel Pharmaco-epidemiology Unit, Clinical Pharmacology & Toxicology, University Hospital Basel), whose methodological and statistical advice I greatly appreciate.

My thanks go also to Rahel Reich (Department of Pharmaceutical Sciences, University of Basel) for her effort concerning her diploma thesis at the Cantonal Hospital of Winterthur.

Furthermore, I wish to express my gratitude to Dr. M. Gabella (Sanofi Aventis Schweiz AG, Meyrin) for the financial support of this dissertation, and I thank Dr. C. Bangerter (e-Mediat AG, Schönbühl) for providing us with the raw data of the drug interaction screening program *Pharmavista*.

I would also like to express my sincere gratitude to Katie Perret (Master of Arts in English and Drama), who spontaneously agreed to proofread my manuscripts.

In addition, I wish to address my thanks to all my colleagues at the Hospital Pharmacy in Baden for the pleasant working atmosphere. I also extend this message to the staff at the Hospital Pharmacy in Winterthur, in particular to Dr. Friedrich Möll.

I wish to express my gratitude to my family and friends for encouragement during my dissertation, with a special thank to my parents.

Finally, I thank Lukas for his love.

## Table of Contents

| | | |
|---|---|---|
| 1 | Abbreviations | 1 |
| 2 | Introduction | 3 |
| 3 | Aims of the Thesis | 11 |
| 4 | Methods, Results and Discussion | 13 |

    Evaluation of frequently used Drug Interaction Screening Programs    15

    Prevalence of Drug-Drug Interactions at Hospital Entry, during Hospital Stay and at Hospital Discharge in a Department of Internal Medicine    41

    Clinical Pharmacist's Intervention to improve the Management of potential Drug-Drug Interactions in a Department of Internal Medicine    67

    Risk Factors for Gastrointestinal Bleeding: a Hospital-based Case-Control Study    89

| | | |
|---|---|---|
| 5 | Conclusions | 109 |

# 1 Abbreviations

| | |
|---|---|
| ABDA | Bundesvereinigung Deutscher Apothekerverbände (Federal organization of the German pharmacist associations) |
| ACE | Angiotensin-converting enzyme |
| ADE | Adverse drug event |
| ADR | Adverse drug reaction |
| ATC | Anatomical therapeutical chemical |
| BMI | Body mass index |
| CD-ROM | Compact disc read-only memory |
| CI | Confidence interval |
| CPOE | Computerized physician order entry |
| CYP | Cytochrome P450 isoenzyme |
| DDI | Drug-drug interaction |
| DIF | Drug Interaction Facts |
| DR | Drug-Reax |
| DRP | Drug-related problem |
| e.g. | For example |
| FPH | Foederatio Pharmaceutica Helvetiae |
| GI | Gastrointestinal |
| H. pylori | Helicobacter pylori |
| ICD-10 | International classification of diseases, $10^{th}$ revision |
| INR | International normalized ratio |
| LI | Lexi-Interact |
| MAO | Monoamine oxidase |
| n | Number of patients |

| | |
|---|---|
| no. | Number |
| NPV | Negative predictive value |
| NRS | Nutrition risk score |
| NSAID | Nonsteroidal antiinflammatory drug |
| OATP | Organic anion transporting polypeptide |
| OR | Odds ratio |
| ORCA | OpeRational ClassificAtion |
| PDA | Personal digital assistant |
| pDDI | Potential drug-drug interaction |
| PPI | Proton pump inhibitor |
| PPV | Positive predictive value |
| PV | Pharmavista |
| SSRI | Selective serotonin reuptake inhibitor |
| VAT | Value-added tax |
| vs | Versus |
| WHO | World Health Organization |
| yr | Year |

## 2  Introduction

Drug-related problems

Besides their beneficial effects, drugs may also induce illness and death. Adverse drug reactions (ADRs) have been the focus in most studies on drug-induced morbidity, but they form only a small part of drug-related problems (DRPs). Medication errors, overdosage, drug dependence, non-compliance and therapeutic failure are further examples of DRPs [1]. Definitions of DRPs are shown in Table I, and the relationships between these terms are given in Figure I.

Table I: Definitions of drug-related problems

| | |
|---|---|
| Drug-related problem | An event or circumstance involving drug therapy that actually or potentially interferes with desired outcomes [2] |
| Medication error | Any error in the process of prescribing, dispensing or administering a drug, whether there are adverse consequences or not [3] |
| Adverse drug reaction | Any response to a drug which is noxious and unintended and which occurs at doses normally used in humans for prophylaxis, diagnosis or therapy of disease, or for the modification of physiological function, given that this noxious response is not due to a medication error [4] |
| Adverse drug event | An injury related to the use of a drug, although the causality of this relationship may not be proven [3] |

Medication errors are defined as problems that involve a mistake in the process from the prescribing to the administration of the drug [3]. Problems that occur even when no errors have been made in the process of drug distribution are called ADRs [4]. Adverse drug events (ADEs) are defined as problems related to the use of a drug, but without evidence of the causality [3].

Despite these definitions, the term "ADR" is used in the literature (e.g. Krahenbuhl-Melcher et al. [5]) – and also in our studies – as a more general term. Consequently, DRPs due to medication errors such as drug-drug interactions (DDIs) are included in the definition of an ADR.

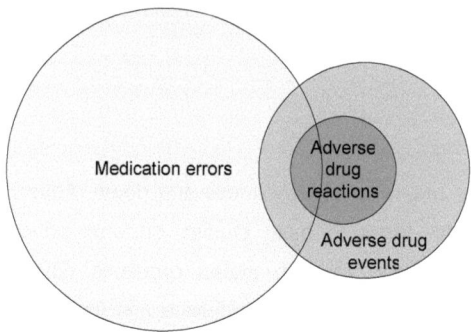

Figure I: Relationship between the terms *medication errors*, *adverse drug reactions* and *adverse drug events* (according to Krahenbuhl-Melcher et al. [5])

Drug-induced morbidity has become a common problem and contributes to a large economic burden for society [6-11]. Classen et al. reported that ADEs significantly prolong the length of hospital stay, increase the costs of treatment, and elevate the risk of death almost two-fold [6]. Some studies suggest that medication errors or ADRs cause between 7'000 and 100'000 deaths annually in the United States [8, 9]. Lazarou et al. reported that ADRs rank between the fourth and sixth leading cause of death in the United States [9].

### Drug-related problems at hospital admission

Hospital admissions associated with ADEs range from 0.2 to 21.7%, of which up to 72% have been judged to be avoidable [12-18]. According to Pirmohamed et al., ADRs (including DDIs) were responsible for 6.5% of hospital admissions. 2.3% of these patients died as a direct result of the ADR [16]. The proportion of ADR-related hospitalizations in a national wide study in The Netherlands was 1.8% of all acute, non-planned hospital admissions [18]. In Switzerland, Lepori et al. showed that 6.4% of the patients presented an ADR at hospital admission, and 65% of these admissions were directly related to an ADR [11].

### Drug-related problems during hospitalization

During a patient's hospital stay, the incidence of ADEs ranges between 0.7 and 6.5%. Up to 57% of these are considered preventable [19-23]. According to Lazarou et al., the overall incidence of serious ADRs in hospitalized patients was 6.7% [9]. Among hospitalized elderly people 61% presented at least one ADR, and an average of 1.7 ADRs per patient was found [17]. According to an analysis of medical inpatients at two Swiss hospitals, in 11% of all hospitalizations clinically relevant ADRs occurred, and the incidence of possibly ADR-related deaths was 0.14% [22].

### Drug-related problems at hospital discharge

Changes in medication at the transition point from outpatient to inpatient care and vice versa may increase the frequency of DRPs [24, 25]. Drug modifications shortly before hospital discharge may be important in this context, because the monitoring of patients significantly declines after hospital discharge [26, 27]. According to Forster et al., 11% of discharged patients developed an ADE within 24 days. 27% of them were preventable. One out of seven injuries was rated as life-threatening [27].

Medication errors

The most common type of avoidable errors during the medication process are prescribing errors [21, 28-30]. According to Bates et al., preventable ADEs occurred mostly at prescribing (56%) and at drug administration (34%), while transcription and dispensing errors occurred at a rate of 6% and 4%, respectively [21]. An investigation on the incidence and clinical significance of prescribing errors in inpatients showed that 54% of prescribing errors were associated with the dosing, and that 61% originated in medication order writing [31]. However, when only serious errors were examined, 58% originated in the prescribing decision [31].

Dean at al. analyzed the reasons of prescribing errors and showed that most mistakes were due to slips in attention, or to prescribers omitting relevant rules. Physicians identified risk factors such as work environment, workload, whether they are prescribing for their own patient, communication within their team, physical and mental well-being, and lack of knowledge. System factors, such as inadequate training, low perceived importance of prescribing, a hierarchical structure of the medical team, and absence of self-awareness were also identified. [32]

## Drug-drug interactions

DDIs occur when the effect of one drug is changed by the presence of another drug. The outcome can be harmful if the DDI causes an increased toxicity of the drug. However, a reduction in therapeutic efficacy due to a DDI may be just as harmful as an increase. For instance, an unintended decrease in anticoagulation by oral anticoagulants is observed when combined with an inducing agent. While such a DDI is unwanted, others can be beneficial and valuable, for instance the co-prescription of antihypertensive drugs and diuretics in order to achieve a better antihypertensive effect. [33]

Epidemiological data relating to the negative clinical outcome of DDIs are rare and therefore we use the expression *potential* (p)DDI. Hamilton et al. pointed out that exposure to pDDIs was associated with a significantly increased risk of hospitalization [34]. According to Pirmohamed et al., one percent of all hospital admissions was caused by DDIs, corresponding to 16% of all patients admitted with ADRs (including DDIs) [16]. In a recent review, an incidence of up to 2.8% of hospital admissions were found to be caused by ADRs due to DDIs [35]. Lepori et al. showed that 21% of all drug-related hospital admissions in a Swiss hospital were caused by DDIs (1.3% of all admissions) [11].

References

1. Johnson JA, Bootman JL. Drug-related morbidity and mortality. A cost-of-illness model. Arch Intern Med 1995 Oct 9; 155 (18): 1949-56.
2. Pharmaceutical Care Network Europe. DRP-classification V5.01 [online]. Available from URL: http://www.pcne.org/dokumenter/PCNE%20classification V501.pdf [Accessed 2007 Jan].
3. Leape LL. Preventing adverse drug events. Am J Health Syst Pharm 1995 Feb 15; 52 (4): 379-82.
4. ASHP guidelines on adverse drug reaction monitoring and reporting. American Society of Hospital Pharmacy. Am J Health Syst Pharm 1995 Feb 15; 52 (4): 417-9.
5. Krahenbuhl-Melcher A, Krahenbuhl S. [Hospital drug safety: medication errors and adverse drug reactions]. Schweiz Rundsch Med Prax 2005 Jun 15; 94 (24-25): 1031-8.
6. Classen DC, Pestotnik SL, Evans RS, et al. Adverse drug events in hospitalized patients. Excess length of stay, extra costs, and attributable mortality. Jama 1997 Jan 22-29; 277 (4): 301-6.
7. Bates DW, Spell N, Cullen DJ, et al. The costs of adverse drug events in hospitalized patients. Adverse Drug Events Prevention Study Group. Jama 1997 Jan 22-29; 277 (4): 307-11.
8. Phillips DP, Christenfeld N, Glynn LM. Increase in US medication-error deaths between 1983 and 1993. Lancet 1998 Feb 28; 351 (9103): 643-4.
9. Lazarou J, Pomeranz BH, Corey PN. Incidence of adverse drug reactions in hospitalized patients: a meta-analysis of prospective studies. Jama 1998 Apr 15; 279 (15): 1200-5.
10. Bates DW. Drugs and adverse drug reactions: how worried should we be? Jama 1998 Apr 15; 279 (15): 1216-7.
11. Lepori V, Perren A, Marone C. [Adverse internal medicine drug effects at hospital admission]. Schweiz Med Wochenschr 1999 Jun 19; 129 (24): 915-22.
12. Hallas J, Haghfelt T, Gram LF, et al. Drug related admissions to a cardiology department; frequency and avoidability. J Intern Med 1990 Oct; 228 (4): 379-84.

13. Einarson TR. Drug-related hospital admissions. Ann Pharmacother 1993 Jul-Aug; 27 (7-8): 832-40.
14. Roughead EE, Gilbert AL, Primrose JG, et al. Drug-related hospital admissions: a review of Australian studies published 1988-1996. Med J Aust 1998 Apr 20; 168 (8): 405-8.
15. Mjorndal T, Boman MD, Hagg S, et al. Adverse drug reactions as a cause for admissions to a department of internal medicine. Pharmacoepidemiol Drug Saf 2002 Jan-Feb; 11 (1): 65-72.
16. Pirmohamed M, James S, Meakin S, et al. Adverse drug reactions as cause of admission to hospital: prospective analysis of 18 820 patients. Bmj 2004 Jul 3; 329 (7456): 15-9.
17. Passarelli MC, Jacob-Filho W, Figueras A. Adverse drug reactions in an elderly hospitalised population: inappropriate prescription is a leading cause. Drugs Aging 2005; 22 (9): 767-77.
18. van der Hooft CS, Sturkenboom MC, van Grootheest K, et al. Adverse drug reaction-related hospitalisations: a nationwide study in The Netherlands. Drug Saf 2006; 29 (2): 161-8.
19. Brennan TA, Leape LL, Laird NM, et al. Incidence of adverse events and negligence in hospitalized patients. Results of the Harvard Medical Practice Study I. N Engl J Med 1991 Feb 7; 324 (6): 370-6.
20. Bates DW, Leape LL, Petrycki S. Incidence and preventability of adverse drug events in hospitalized adults. J Gen Intern Med 1993 Jun; 8 (6): 289-94.
21. Bates DW, Cullen DJ, Laird N, et al. Incidence of adverse drug events and potential adverse drug events. Implications for prevention. ADE Prevention Study Group. Jama 1995 Jul 5; 274 (1): 29-34.
22. Fattinger K, Roos M, Vergeres P, et al. Epidemiology of drug exposure and adverse drug reactions in two swiss departments of internal medicine. Br J Clin Pharmacol 2000 Feb; 49 (2): 158-67.
23. Thomas EJ, Studdert DM, Burstin HR, et al. Incidence and types of adverse events and negligent care in Utah and Colorado. Med Care 2000 Mar; 38 (3): 261-71.
24. Himmel W, Tabache M, Kochen MM. What happens to long-term medication when general practice patients are referred to hospital? Eur J Clin Pharmacol 1996; 50 (4): 253-7.

25. Smith L, McGowan L, Moss-Barclay C, et al. An investigation of hospital generated pharmaceutical care when patients are discharged home from hospital. Br J Clin Pharmacol 1997 Aug; 44 (2): 163-5.
26. Cook RI, Render M, Woods DD. Gaps in the continuity of care and progress on patient safety. Bmj 2000 Mar 18; 320 (7237): 791-4.
27. Forster AJ, Murff HJ, Peterson JF, et al. Adverse drug events occurring following hospital discharge. J Gen Intern Med 2005 Apr; 20 (4): 317-23.
28. Leape LL, Bates DW, Cullen DJ, et al. Systems analysis of adverse drug events. ADE Prevention Study Group. Jama 1995 Jul 5; 274 (1): 35-43.
29. Fijn R, Van den Bemt PM, Chow M, et al. Hospital prescribing errors: epidemiological assessment of predictors. Br J Clin Pharmacol 2002 Mar; 53 (3): 326-31.
30. Lisby M, Nielsen LP, Mainz J. Errors in the medication process: frequency, type, and potential clinical consequences. Int J Qual Health Care 2005 Feb; 17 (1): 15-22.
31. Dean B, Schachter M, Vincent C, et al. Prescribing errors in hospital inpatients: their incidence and clinical significance. Qual Saf Health Care 2002 Dec; 11 (4): 340-4.
32. Dean B, Schachter M, Vincent C, et al. Causes of prescribing errors in hospital inpatients: a prospective study. Lancet 2002 Apr 20; 359 (9315): 1373-8.
33. Stockley IH, editor. Stockley's drug interactions. 6th ed. London, Chicago: The Pharmaceutical Press; 2002.
34. Hamilton RA, Briceland LL, Andritz MH. Frequency of hospitalization after exposure to known drug-drug interactions in a Medicaid population. Pharmacotherapy 1998 Sep-Oct; 18 (5): 1112-20.
35. Jankel CA, Fitterman LK. Epidemiology of drug-drug interactions as a cause of hospital admissions. Drug Saf 1993 Jul; 9 (1): 51-9.

# 3 Aims of the Thesis

The general aim of this thesis was to elucidate the importance of potential drug-drug interactions (pDDIs) as a contributing factor in drug safety issues.

The first focus of this thesis was an evaluation study of frequently used drug interaction screening programs. The specific objective of this study was to critically appraise these programs regarding their possible implementation in the Medical Department of the Cantonal Hospital of Baden.

The second focus of this thesis was to identify clinically relevant pDDIs in the Medical Department of the Cantonal Hospital of Baden, with the goal of improving the clinical management of pDDIs by pharmacist interventions during hospitalization and at hospital discharge.

The third focus of this thesis was to investigate risk factors for gastrointestinal bleeding possibly leading to hospital admission and to assess the role of pDDIs as a cause of this adverse drug reaction.

## 4 Methods, Results and Discussion

The content of this dissertation is the subject of four publications. Thus, the following pages contain these papers starting with the evaluation of drug interaction screening programs, continuing with the prevalence of drug-drug interactions during hospitalization and the pharmacist intervention study and ending with a case-control study about risk factors for gastrointestinal bleeding.

# Evaluation of frequently used Drug Interaction Screening Programs

Priska Vonbach[1], André Dubied[1], Stephan Krähenbühl[2], Jürg H Beer[3]

1 Hospital Pharmacy, Cantonal Hospital of Baden, Switzerland

2 Clinical Pharmacology & Toxicology, University Hospital Basel, Switzerland

3 Department of Medicine, Cantonal Hospital of Baden, Switzerland

## Abstract

Introduction
Drug interaction screening programs are an important tool to check prescriptions of multiple drugs for potential drug-drug interactions (pDDIs). Several programs are available on the market. They differ in layout, update frequency, search functions, content and price. The aim of the current study was to critically appraise several interaction screening programs in the Department of Medicine of a Swiss public teaching hospital.

Methods
A drug interaction screening program had to fulfil minimal requirements (information on effect, severity rating, clinical management, mechanism and literature) in order to be admitted to the present evaluation. The 100 most frequently used drugs in the Cantonal Hospital of Baden, Switzerland, were used to test the comprehensiveness of the programs. Qualitative criteria were used for the assessment of the drug interaction monographs. In a precision analysis, 30 drugs with and 30 drugs without pDDIs of clinical importance were tested. In addition, 16 typical patient profiles were checked for pDDIs, using *Stockley's Drug Interactions* as a reference.

Results
Out of nine programs included, the following four fulfilled the above mentioned criteria: *Drug Interaction Facts*, *Drug-Reax*, *Lexi-Interact* and *Pharmavista*. *Drug Interaction Facts* contained the lowest number of drugs and was therefore the least qualified program. *Lexi-Interact* condenses many DDIs into one group, resulting in less specific information, whereas *Pharmavista* and *Drug-Reax* offer excellent interaction monographs. In the precision analysis, *Lexi-Interact* showed the best sensitivity (1.00), followed by *Drug-Reax* and *Pharmavista* (0.83 each) and *Drug Interaction Facts* (0.63). The analysis of patient profiles revealed that out of 157 pDDIs found by all programs, only 18 (11%) were detected by all of them. No program found more than 50% of the total number of pDDIs. A further evaluation using *Stockley's Drug Interactions* as the gold standard revealed that *Pharmavista* achieved a sensitivity of 0.86 (versus *Drug Interaction Facts*, *Lexi-Interact* and

*Drug-Reax* with a sensitivity of 0.71 each) with an acceptable positive predictive value of 0.67.

Conclusion

In order to detect most pDDIs without causing too many false positive results, drug interaction screening programs should have a high sensitivity and a high positive predictive value. *Pharmavista* offers the highest sensitivity of the programs evaluated with a positive predictive value in an acceptable range. An increase in sensitivity is possible by the combination of two programs.

## Introduction

Adverse drug reactions are associated with considerable morbidity and mortality [1, 2]. For instance, they are responsible for up to 5% of hospital admissions. According to a recently published study one percent of all hospital admissions were caused by drug-drug interactions (DDIs), corresponding to 16% of all patients admitted with adverse drug reactions [3]. In fact, the clinical outcome of a potential (p)DDI is often unknown, and epidemiological data are rare. Juurlink et al. calculated odds ratios of 6.6 for hypoglycaemia in patients treated with glyburide in combination with co-trimoxazole, 11.7 for digoxin toxicity in patients treated with clarithromycin and 20.3 for hyperkalaemia in patients with angiotensin-converting enzyme inhibitors combined with potassium-sparing diuretics [4].

In order to reduce the number and to improve the management of pDDIs, physicians primarily have to be aware of the presence of a pDDI. Recommendations include different books, tables and consultation of the primary literature. An automatically applied drug interaction screening program would be highly desirable and timesaving for the drug prescription.

Different studies evaluating such programs have been conducted and published before [5-8]. Hazlet et al. focused on the precision analysis of nine non identified drug interaction screening programs. Sensitivity, specificity, positive (PPV) and negative predictive value (NPV) were determined by the analysis of 16 pDDIs contained within six patient profiles [6]. Jankel and Martin evaluated six widely used drug interaction screening programs according to criteria developed by a panel of seven pharmacists. The panel determined that a drug interaction screening program should be user friendly and efficient, provide guidance in making a decision to intervene and be relevant to the user's practice. Additional criteria fell into three categories: knowledge base, presentation of the information as well as hardware and software attributes. None of the six evaluated programs was considered to be ideal by the panel [5]. Barla et al. listed nine criteria to test the scientific quality of drug interaction screening programs. Drug pairs with or without interactions have been selected for each of these criteria and have been used for the evaluation of eight programs. None of these programs was considered to be satisfactory [9]. Barrons studied the accuracy, comprehensiveness and user friendliness of nine drug interaction screening programs running on personal digital assistants (PDA). Accuracy was scored by the summation of software sensitivity, specificity, PPV and NPV. The comprehensiveness of each program was determined by the number of components provided in the drug interaction monograph. The time to find out the management of five important pDDIs defined each program's ease of use. The aggregate scores for accuracy, comprehensiveness and ease of use were calculated [7]. Perrin et al. evaluated seven drug interaction screening programs on the basis of 60 common pDDIs in hospitalized patients, 40 pDDIs in ambulatory patients, 10 classical and well-known pDDIs and 10 recently discovered pDDIs. In addition to the detection of the mentioned pDDIs, the program's assessment included information on the severity, the mechanism, the symptoms, the clinical management of the pDDIs and on the references provided. Update frequency, language, price, installation, print-out of the summary, user friendliness and connections to the patient's record were also decisive criteria [8].

None of the mentioned evaluation studies fulfilled our requirements, however. Two studies [5, 9] were conducted in 1992 and were judged not to be actual. One evaluation did not mention the program's names [6] and Barrons study [7] focused on PDA programs only. The latest study [8] was published when the present evaluation was in progress and is going to be discussed at the end of this evaluation.

The specific aim of our study was to critically appraise frequently used drug interaction screening programs regarding a possible implementation in the Department of Medicine of a Swiss public teaching hospital.

## Methods

Inclusion criteria

Nine different computerized drug interaction screening programs (British National Formulary, Drug Interaction Facts, Drug-Reax, ePocrates MultiCheck, Lexi-Interact, Pharmavista, Stockley's Drug Interactions, The Medical Letter and Vidal) were initially included in our evaluation. In order to be admitted to the final evaluation (see below), an interaction screening program had to fulfil several minimal requirements: information in the interaction monographs on the effect (pharmacokinetic and/or pharmacodynamic) of a specific pDDI, on the clinical management and on the mechanism of the pDDI and about the references provided regarding this pDDI. Furthermore, a severity rating was required.

Only four out of the nine drug interaction screening programs included fulfilled all of these criteria and were chosen for the additional studies as detailed below.

Qualitative assessment of the drug interaction monographs

To assess the quality of the drug interaction monographs, eight pDDIs were analyzed with each program: carbamazepine - acetaminophen, lamotrigine - valproic acid, indinavir - St. John's wort, simvastatin - voriconazole, aspirin - enalapril, potassium chloride - spironolactone, isosorbide dinitrate - sildenafil and dihydroergotamine - sumatriptan. All of these pDDIs were classified as *major* or *moderate* by any of the inspected drug interaction screening programs.

Different questions had to be answered: How useful is the information on the effect, the clinical management and the mechanism of the pDDI? How complete is the literature provided? Do programs perform drug grouping according to their therapeutical group and/or pharmacokinetics? And if so, is the categorisation useful? Are there other ratings than those about the severity of the adverse reaction? Does a documentation rating exist? Is there information about the onset of the effect? Is there a standardization concerning the severity rating, the documentation rating and the onset of the effect? Is the content of the monographs supported by the literature cited? If a question could not be answered with the available information, the editors of the program were contacted.

## Comprehensiveness of the drug lists in the interaction screening programs

In this part of the final evaluation, we investigated the completeness of the drug interaction screening programs concerning drugs. Programs were screened for the 100 most frequently prescribed drugs in the Department of Medicine of the Cantonal Hospital of Baden, Switzerland, in 2003. The frequency of the drug prescriptions was calculated as therapeutical days using the Defined Daily Dose as defined by the WHO [10]. If a drug name was not found by the drug interaction screening program, other nomenclatures – not familiar for European users – were tested using the *Martindale* [11].

Precision analysis

The performance of the drug interaction screening programs was assessed for sensitivity[i], specificity[ii], PPV[iii] and NPV[iv]. Sensitivity was defined as the ability of the drug interaction screening program to correctly identify pDDIs that were clinically important. Specificity was defined as the ability of the drug interaction screening program to ignore interactions that were clinically unimportant. The PPV indicated the probability that, when the drug interaction screening program identified a pDDI, it was a pDDI defined as clinically important. The NPV indicated the probability that a pDDI was defined as clinically unimportant, if the drug interaction screening program ignored the pDDI. [12]

A total of 60 drug pairs (Table I) were selected using the hard copy of *Stockley's Drug Interactions* [13], which was defined as the gold standard. Thirty drug pairs were labelled as clinical important (*Stockley* defined the interaction as *clinically important* and/or a monitoring was required), and 30 pairs were labelled as *clinically unimportant* (*Stockley* defined the interaction as *clinically unimportant* and/or *no effect* was observed). Furthermore, all of the inspected drugs had to be included in every drug interaction screening program evaluated.

---

i Sensitivity: The ability to detect clinically important interactions. Sensitivity = number of true-positives / (number of true-positives + number of false-negatives)
ii Specificity: The ability to ignore clinically unimportant interactions. Specificity = number of true-negatives / (number of true-negatives + number of false-positives)
iii Positive predictive value (PPV): When a drug interaction is found, the probability that the interaction is clinically important. PPV = number of true-positives / (number of true-positives + number of false-positives)
iv Negative predictive value (NPV): When a drug interaction is ignored, the probability that the interaction is clinically unimportant. NPV = number of true-negatives / (number of true-negatives + number of false-negatives)

Table I: Drug pairs included in the precison analysis. Thirty clinically important and 30 clinically unimportant potential drug-drug interactions were chosen using *Stockley's Drug Interactions* as a reference.

| clinically important interactions | clinically unimportant interactions |
|---|---|
| alprazolam - digoxin | acyclovir - cyclosporine |
| amiodarone - clarithromycin | allopurinol - atenolol |
| antacids/iron - levofloxacin | allopurinol - digoxin |
| captopril - lithium | aspirin - digoxin |
| carbamazepine - felodipine | atenolol - eletriptan |
| chlorpromazine - haloperidol | azithromycin - triazolam |
| cimetidine - vardenafil | busulfan - fluconazole |
| ciprofloxacin - theophylline | candesartan - digoxin |
| cisplatin - gentamicin | cefotaxime - ofloxacin |
| clarithromycin - triazolam | ciprofloxacin - oral contraceptive |
| clindamycin - gentamicin | clonidine - maprotiline |
| clonidine - imipramine | caffeine - grapefruit juice |
| clozapine - fluvoxamine | co-trimoxazole - indinavir |
| cyclosporine - enalapril | dexamethasone - theophylline |
| desipramine - ritonavir | didanosine - fluconazole |
| dexamethasone - itraconazole | diltiazem - pravastatin |
| digoxin - diltiazem | doxorubicin - tamoxifen |
| digoxin - telmisartan | enalapril - sildenafil |
| dihydroergotamine - eletriptan | ethinylestradiol - orlistat |
| diltiazem - lovastatin | flurazepam - warfarin |
| diltiazem - rifampicin | gentamicin - lincomycin |
| disulfiram - metronidazole | grapefruit juice - pravastatin |
| droperidol - sotalol | haloperidol - valproic acid |
| ergotamine - erythromycin | imipramine - olanzapine |
| felodipine - itraconazole | lidocaine - verapamil |
| furosemide - indometacin | lithium - olanzapine |
| ganciclovir - lamivudine | methotrexate - tacrolimus |
| moxifloxacin - thioridazine | metronidazole - sucralfate |
| orale contraceptive - rifampicin | metronidazole - sulfasalazine |
| penicillin - probenecid | ofloxacin - theophylline |

If a program detected a specific DDI, which was not listed by *Stockley*, the literature cited by the program was checked concerning the year of publication. If the references cited were between 2002 and 2004, they had to be reassessed, because the last edition of *Stockley* was published in 2002. The clinical relevance of such DDIs was judged by a clinical pharmacist and by a physician.

Patient profiles

This final part of the study evaluated the clinical practicability of the programs. Sixteen patients with different diagnoses were chosen and their drug lists were analyzed for pDDIs. Potential DDIs were arranged regarding the severity rating (*major*, *moderate* or *minor*). For *Pharmavista*, the lowest three levels of five severity ratings were condensed into one to simplify the levels.

The clinically relevant DDIs identified were then compared with *Stockley's Drug Interactions* [13], which was again used as the gold standard. Sensitivity, specificity, PPV and NPV were calculated for each program, identically as described above for the precision analysis. If a drug was not included in *Stockley*, the corresponding drug pairs were excluded from the analysis. DDIs detected by the programs but not listed in *Stockley* were considered to be false positive results. If such DDIs had been published after the year 2001, they were reassessed. If they were considered to be clinically important, they were accepted as a positive result. Otherwise, they were considered as a false positive result.

## Results

Four drug interaction screening programs (*Drug Interaction Facts* (DIF), *Drug-Reax* (DR), *Lexi-Interact* (LI) and *Pharmavista* (PV)) fulfilled the mentioned inclusion criteria. These programs are described in more detail in Table II. In all of these programs, the interaction monographs are divided into different chapters for severity, effects, mechanism, clinical management, discussion (or summary) and literature. As an exception, in LI the effect and the mechanism are provided in a common chapter called *summary*.

Table II: Characterisation of the drug interaction screening programs included in the final analysis

| Program / Homepage | Editor / Data source | Version | Update frequency | Price[a] | Version used in this study / Date |
|---|---|---|---|---|---|
| Drug Interaction Facts http://www.factsandcomparisons.com | Tatro DS / eFacts / Facts & Comparisons | online | monthly | $ 473[b] | online Mars - June 2004 |
|  |  | CD-ROM | every 3 months | $ 199 |  |
|  |  | PDA | every 3 months | $ 69 |  |
| Drug-Reax http://www.micromedex.com | Thomson MICROMEDEX | online | every 3 months | € 695 | CD-ROM Vol. 119, 120, 121 |
|  |  | CD-ROM | every 3 months | € 634 |  |
|  |  | PDA | every 3 months | € 99 |  |
| Lexi-Interact http://www.lexi.com | Lexi-Comp | online | daily | $ 425[c] | online Mars - June 2004 |
|  |  | CD-ROM | monthly | $ 475[d] |  |
|  |  | PDA | monthly | $ 75 |  |
| Pharmavista http://www.pharmavista.ch | e-Mediat AG / ABDA-Datenbank | online | monthly | CHF 650[e] | online Mars - June 2004 |
|  |  | CD-ROM | monthly |  |  |
|  |  | PDA | every 3 months | CHF 120 |  |

a) Prices for a subscription for one year, single user, exclusive VAT, August 2005
b) Price for the whole database *eFacts*, interaction module not available separately
c) Price for *Lexi-Comp OnLine* (13 databases), inclusive *Lexi-Comp Complete* PDA-version (15 databases), *Lexi-Interact* not available separately
d) Price for *Lexi-Comp Complete* (15 databases), inclusive online and PDA-version, *Lexi-Interact* not available separately
e) Price for the whole database *Pharmavista* for four users, online and CD-ROM version together, interaction module not available separately

ABDA = Bundesvereinigung Deutscher Apothekerverbände (federal organization of the German pharmacist associations), CD-ROM = compact disc ready-only memory, PDA = personal digital assistant, VAT = value-added tax

## Qualitative assessment of the drug interaction monographs

All drug interaction screening programs offered useful information on the effect, the clinical management and the mechanism of the pDDI, and the literature. However, PV's and DR's monographs are of excellent quality (detailed and sophisticated) and were assessed as superior compared to the other two programs. As described above, LI does not provide a separate chapter concerning the effect and the mechanism of the pDDI.

Each of the four programs sometimes concentrated similar drugs into one monograph, but to a different extent. DR rarely pooled more than two interacting drugs. The grouping of similar drugs in terms of therapeutical effects and pharmacokinetics by DIF and PV was considered to be user-friendly (e.g. potassium salts - potassium-sparing diuretics or nitrates - phosphodiesterase-5 inhibitors). However in LI, the condensation of individual drugs into drug classes was done in an excessive manner. This concept therefore resulted in less specific information within the monograph of a specific drug. For example, the interaction between simvastatin and voriconazole appeared in the monograph *CYP3A4 substrates - CYP3A4 inhibitors (moderate)*, and no information about increased simvastatin plasma concentrations and possible rhabdomyolysis or about alternative drugs like pravastatin or fluvastatin were given. The same problem occurred regarding the pDDI between dihydroergotamine and sumatriptan, which was displayed in the monograph *Serotonin Modulators - Serotonin Modulators* together with another 50 drugs called *Serotonin Modulators*. As a consequence, no precise information on the effect and the clinical management of individual pDDIs were available.

In addition to the severity rating, LI offered a classification called *risk rating*, where not only the severity, but also the clinical management is taken into account. DIF provided a second classification as well. The so-called *significance level* represents a mixture between the rating of the severity and the documentation of the pDDI in the literature. Documentation ratings were provided by all four programs evaluated.

The onset of the effect was mentioned separately in the monographs of DIF and DR and sometimes also in LI. No separate chapter existed in PV, but the onset of the effect was usually mentioned in the description of the effect.

Severity ratings (as well as the *risk rating* and the *significance level*), documentation ratings and information on the onset of the effect were standardized by each program.

Citations in DIF, DR and LI were clearly linked with the corresponding literature. Regrettably, in PV the references were not assigned to specific statements in the monograph.

<u>Comprehensiveness of the drug lists in the interaction screening programs</u>

Figure I shows the number of drugs not included in the drug interaction screening programs and the number of drugs with an unusual nomenclature for European users. The number of drugs not included in the respective program was highest for DIF (25% of all drugs tested) and lowest for LI (3% of all drugs tested). To give some examples for an unusual nomenclature in Europe: acetaminophen instead of paracetamol, albuterol instead of salbutamol or torsemide instead of torasemide.

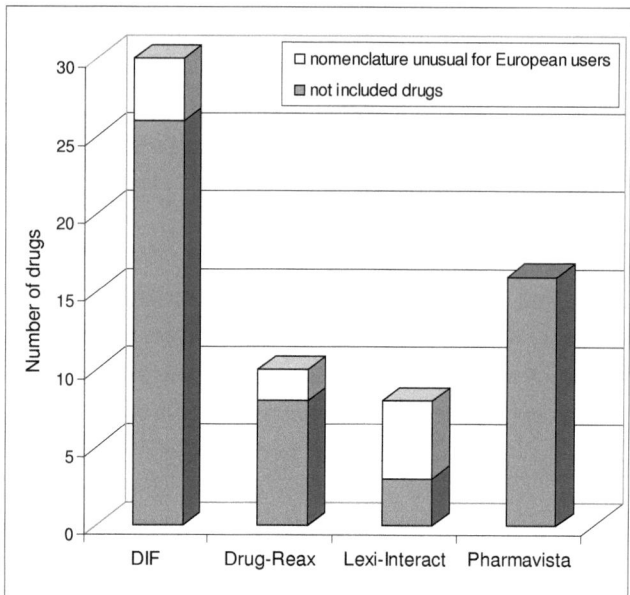

Figure I: Comprehensiveness of the drug interaction screening programs regarding the drugs included. The programs were tested for the comprehensiveness of their drug lists by checking the 100 drugs used most often on the medical wards of the Cantonal Hospital of Baden, Switzerland, in the year 2003. The figure shows the number of drugs not recognized by the drug interaction screening programs and the number of drugs with an unusual nomenclature for European users.
DIF = Drug Interaction Facts

## Precision analysis

LI showed the best sensitivity, followed by DR and PV (Table III). Both DR and PV failed to detect five DDIs, whereas DIF found only two thirds of clinically important pDDIs.

Table III: Results of the precison analysis. Thirty clinically important and 30 clinically unimportant potential drug-drug interactions (see Table I) were analyzed.

|  | DIF | DR | LI | PV |
|---|---|---|---|---|
| True positive | 19 | 25 | 30 | 25 |
| False positive | 0 | 3 | 6 | 5 |
| True negative | 30 | 27 | 24 | 25 |
| False negative | 11 | 5 | 0 | 5 |
| Sensitivity | 0.63 | 0.83 | 1.00 | 0.83 |
| Specificity | 1.00 | 0.90 | 0.80 | 0.83 |
| Positive predictive value | 1.00 | 0.89 | 0.83 | 0.83 |
| Negative predictive value | 0.73 | 0.84 | 1.00 | 0.83 |

DIF = Drug Interaction Facts, DR = Drug-Reax, LI = Lexi-Interact, PV = Pharmavista

False positive results were provided by DR (3), LI (6) and PV (5). The cited literature has generally been published before 2002, with four exceptions. In the monograph of lithium - olanzapine, DR referred to a product information of 2002 [14]. Regarding the drug pair theophylline - ofloxacin, PV referred to a product information of 2004 [15], and concerning the fluconazole - busulfan and verapamil - lidocaine interactions, LI referred to a recent publication of in vitro and in vivo studies [16]. These pDDIs were reassessed and found to be clinically unimportant.

Patient profiles

The medication profiles of 16 medical patients, who were treated by a mean number of 15 ± 6 drugs, were analyzed. Totally, 99 different drugs were prescribed and 1'376 different drug pairs had to be tested. As shown in Figure II, the number of pDDIs detected with *minor* and *moderate* severity was comparable between the programs. In contrast, regarding the pDDIs with *major* severity, the number detected by DR was 34, whereas the other programs detected only two to four of such pDDIs. A closer look at the pDDIs with *major* severity detected by DR revealed that 18 out of the 34 pDDIs were caused by interactions between valerian preparations and so-called hepatotoxic drugs. These pDDIs were not listed by the other programs. The total number of the pDDIs detected was 157, and the number of the pDDIs detected by all programs was 18. The discrepancy between these figures suggests that there are large differences in the pDDIs identified by the programs.

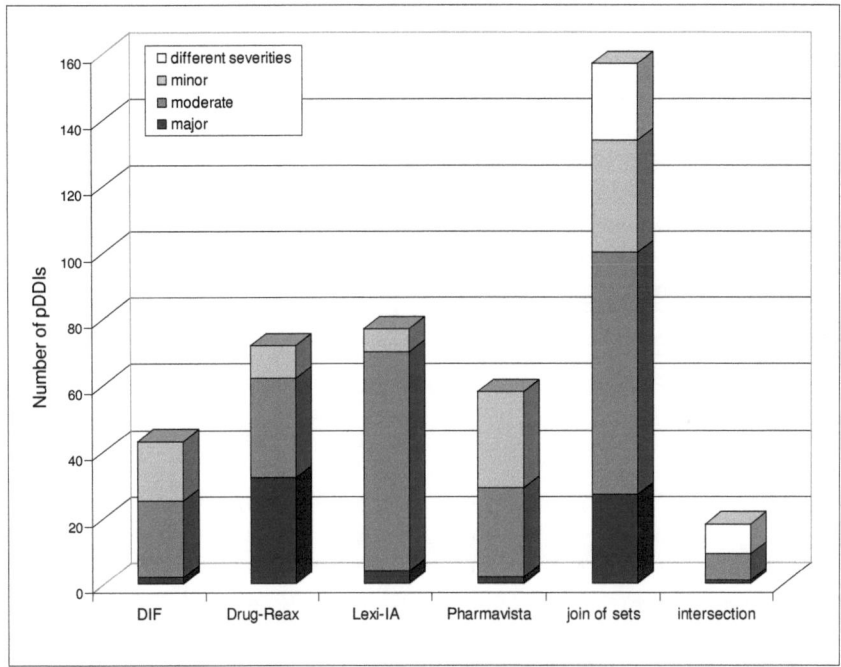

Figure II: Detection of potential drug-drug interactions (pDDIs) by different drug interaction screening programs. The drug profiles of 16 medical patients of the Cantonal Hospital of Baden, Switzerland, were analyzed. The patients were treated with an average number of 15 ± 6 drugs, resulting in a total of 1'070 different drug pairs to be analyzed. Different severities means that the pDDI is categorised into different severities by several programs.
DIF = Drug Interaction Facts, Lexi-IA = Lexi-Interact;

In order to perform a precision analysis with clinical relevance, *Stockley's Drug Interactions* was used as the gold standard. Out of the 99 different drugs used by the patients, *Stockley* did not include eight, which were therefore excluded. In addition, 26 drug pairs could not be assessed clearly for different reasons and were therefore also excluded. Finally, 951 drug pairs were assessed whereof 35 clinically relevant pDDIs were detected using *Stockley*. Taken together, a total of 74 additional pDDIs were detected by the four drug interaction screening programs. These 74 pDDIs were reassessed regarding their date of publication. Two of them, published after 2002, were found to be clinically relevant and were accepted as positive results, whereas the remaining 72 pDDIs were considered to be false positive results. As shown in Table IV, all drug interaction screening programs showed high specificities (≥ 0.95) and also high NPV (0.99). In comparison, the sensitivities were lower (0.71 - 0.86), as well as the PPV (ranging from 0.36 for LI to 0.69 for DIF).

Table IV: Analysis of patient profiles. Drug profiles of 16 patients from the Cantonal Hospital of Baden, Switzerland, were analyzed for potential drug-drug interactions. The patients were treated with 15 ± 6 drugs, resulting in a total of 1'376 different drug pairs. Of these, 951 could finally be analyzed. For most of the drug pairs excluded, one of the drugs was not listed in *Stockley's Drug Interactions*, which was used as the reference.

|  | DIF | DR | LI | PV |
|---|---|---|---|---|
| True positive | 25 | 25 | 25 | 30 |
| False positive | 11 | 16 | 46 | 15 |
| True negative | 905 | 900 | 870 | 901 |
| False negative | 10 | 10 | 10 | 5 |
| Sensitivity | 0.71 | 0.71 | 0.71 | 0.86 |
| Specificity | 0.99 | 0.98 | 0.95 | 0.98 |
| Positive predictive value | 0.69 | 0.61 | 0.36 | 0.67 |
| Negative predictive value | 0.99 | 0.99 | 0.99 | 0.99 |

DIF = Drug Interaction Facts, DR = Drug-Reax, LI = Lexi-Interact, PV = Pharmavista

## Discussion

Drug interaction screening programs vary in price, update frequencies, search and filter functions, and in the information within the interaction monographs. The comparison of prices is of limited usefulness, however, because different packages are included and drug interaction screening programs are often not available separated from other programs. The information provided within the interaction monographs ranges from a short comment on the effect and the clinical management to detailed descriptions regarding the effect and its onset, the severity, the mechanism, the clinical management, documentation rating, discussion and literature.

Unavailable severity rating (*ePocrates MultiCheck*, *Stockley's Drug Interactions* and *The Medical Letter*), non existing description of the mechanism (*British National Formulary* and *ePocrates MultiCheck*) and lacking declaration of literature (*British National Formulary*, *ePocrates MultiCheck* and *Vidal*) were reasons for not fulfilling the inclusion criteria. Thus, only four drug interaction screening programs (DIF, DR, LI and PV) could be included into the final evaluation.

<u>Qualitative assessment of the drug interaction monographs</u>
The condensation of different drugs into one drug interaction monograph appears to be acceptable, if the same type of pDDI is documented or can be expected, and if the clinical management is identical. In DIF and PV, the grouping of drugs was done to a reasonable extent, whereas DR rarely condensed drugs into groups. In contrast, LI partially condensed drugs into large groups, reducing the information about individual pDDIs and making it difficult to identify individual drugs. Concerning LI, the drug groups formed were often too large and more drug-specific information would be desirable.

Concerning the severity rating, more than three levels (e.g. *major, moderate, minor*) do not appear to be clinically meaningful. A *significance level* (DIF), which combines the severity of a pDDI with its documentation, may not be helpful or may even be misleading. The criteria for level four (the second lowest level) in DIF are as follows: *Interaction may cause moderate-to-major effects; data are very limited*. Even if the documentation is scarce, severe complications may develop. However, on this level, the user may tend not to consider such a DDI to be potentially serious.

On the other hand, the *risk rating* concept offered by LI appears to be an interesting approach. The *risk rating* is based on the OpeRational ClassificAtion (ORCA) system [17]. The ORCA system takes into account the potential severity of the adverse drug reaction due to the pDDI, the factors known to increase or decrease the risk for an adverse drug reaction and the existing management alternatives to avoid the pDDI or to reduce the risk for an adverse drug reaction by other means.

Comprehensiveness of the drug lists in the interaction screening programs
Regarding the comprehensiveness of the drug lists covered by the programs, DIF found only three quarters out of the 100 most frequently prescribed drugs in the Medical Clinic of a Cantonal Hospital in Switzerland. On the other hand, LI missed only three out of the 100 drugs tested, out of which two are not registered in the United States (metamizol and phenprocoumon) [18] and one is probably unimportant concerning pDDIs (fig sirup). PV, the only European program, surprisingly missed 16 drugs. However, also in this case, the missed drugs were mostly considered not to be important regarding clinically relevant pDDIs. On the other hand, the confidence of the user into the program will decrease, when drugs are frequently not included, even if the pDDIs associated with these drugs are of only minor clinical importance.

Precision analysis
A good drug interaction screening program should be able to detect clinically important pDDIs (high sensitivity). Regarding safety, false negative results (not detected pDDIs) are clinically more important than false positive results. Nevertheless, if the PPV is too low, there will be many unnecessary alerts, which may discourage the user, who may therefore miss clinically important pDDIs [19-21].

In our precision analysis, LI showed the best sensitivity (1.00), followed by DR and PV (0.83 each) and DIF (0.63). These values compare well with other studies, which revealed sensitivities from 0.87 to 1.00 [7] and from 0.44 to 0.88 [6].

The selection of the drug pairs in the study of Barrons [7] needs to be appraised critically. In this study, three programs were chosen as a reference, whereof two originated from the same editor as the evaluated PDA programs (*iFacts* - DIF and

*Mobile Micromedex* - DR). The PDA programs were therefore assessed on the basis of their own full versions. As a consequence, regarding sensitivity, *iFacts* and *Mobile Micromedex* may have performed better in Barron's evaluation than in our study (the sensitivities were 0.98 vs 0.63 for DIF and 0.95 vs 0.83 for DR in Barron's vs our study). In order to avoid such biases, we used *Stockley's Drug Interactions* [13] as a reference in our study.

Patient profiles

The analysis of the patient profiles included an assessment of the pDDIs identified by each program and a comparison with *Stockley's Drug Interactions*, which was again used as a reference.

Taken together, the programs identified a total of 157 pDDIs within the 1'376 drug pairs examined, whereby none of the drug interaction screening programs detected more then a half of the pDDIs. Only 18 of these pDDIs (11% of the total) were detected by all programs. The number of drugs not included in the programs (DIF 19, DR 8, LI 8 and PV 10) cannot fully explain these findings. The interaction between valerian and hepatotoxic drugs, which revealed 18 potentially severe DDIs only listed in DR, offers an additional explanation for this discrepancy between the programs. The clinical significance of these interactions can be questioned, however. In the referenced study [22], four cases with liver toxicity related to the use of an herbal product containing valerian and skullcap are presented. The authors of this study concluded that valerian should not be combined with other herbs with the potential to cause hepatotoxicity. A review of the literature [23-31] revealed no information about hepatotoxic effects of valerian or about an increased risk for hepatotoxicity when valerian is combined with hepatotoxic drugs. Inclusion of pDDIs with questionable clinical significance offers therefore an additional explanation for the observed differences between the drug interaction screening programs tested.

When the patient profiles were analyzed with *Stockley* as a reference, the programs did not differ much in their sensitivity (range 0.71 - 0.86) or NPV (0.99), but in the PPV (range 0.36 - 0.67). The lowest PPV was found for LI, which achieved its sensitivity (0.71) on the cost of a low PPV (0.36). In other words, the probability that a pDDI detected by LI is clinically important equals only 36%, a value appearing to be too low. In comparison to the precision analysis, the results from the analysis of the patient profiles were not always matching. For example, LI achieved good results in the precision analysis (sensitivity 1.00, PPV 0.83), but scored quite badly regarding the patient profiles (sensitivity 0.71, PPV 0.36). In contrast, PV (0.86 vs 0.83) and DIF (0.71 vs 0.63) performed better with regard to sensitivity in the analysis of the patient profiles as compared to the precision analysis. Possibilities to explain these discrepancies include the number of drug pairs analyzed, the ratio between drug pairs with and without interaction (1:1 in the precision analysis and 35:916 in the analysis of the patient profiles), and the drugs analyzed. The patient profiles offer a better reflection of the real situation than the drugs chosen in the precision analysis.

## Comparison of the current with other studies

Perrin et al. [8] evaluated seven drug interaction screening programs on the basis of 60 common pDDIs observed in hospitalized patients, 40 pDDIs in ambulant patients, 10 classic and well-known pDDIs and 10 only recently established pDDIs. Regrettably, the authors gave no information about the reference used for comparison. According to this study, *Thériaque*, *The Medical Letter* and DR showed the best performance. The authors also noticed that PV could be the best drug interaction screening program, if it detected more pDDIs (problem of low sensitivity). Unfortunately, PV does not link well drug names in German, potentially leading to false negative results. If the user enters trade names or the Latin denomination, much more pDDIs can be detected.

## Conclusion

In order to detect clinically important pDDIs within a reasonable time, we propose to use a program with a high sensitivity, a high NPV and an acceptable PPV. Among the programs tested, PV offers the highest sensitivity, a high NPV and also an acceptable PPV, and can therefore be recommended. An increase in the sensitivity could be achieved by the combination of two drug interaction screening programs. Considering PV, possible improvements include the correct linking of drug names, a more precise linking of the references to the text in the monographs, an enlargement of the drug list and an edition in English.

**References**

1. Einarson TR. Drug-related hospital admissions. Ann Pharmacother 1993 Jul-Aug; 27 (7-8): 832-40.
2. Lazarou J, Pomeranz BH, Corey PN. Incidence of adverse drug reactions in hospitalized patients: a meta-analysis of prospective studies. Jama 1998 Apr 15; 279 (15): 1200-5.
3. Pirmohamed M, James S, Meakin S, et al. Adverse drug reactions as cause of admission to hospital: prospective analysis of 18 820 patients. Bmj 2004 Jul 3; 329 (7456): 15-9.
4. Juurlink DN, Mamdani M, Kopp A, et al. Drug-drug interactions among elderly patients hospitalized for drug toxicity. Jama 2003 Apr 2; 289 (13): 1652-8.
5. Jankel CA, Martin BC. Evaluation of six computerized drug interaction screening programs. Am J Hosp Pharm 1992 Jun; 49 (6): 1430-5.
6. Hazlet TK, Lee TA, Hansten PD, et al. Performance of community pharmacy drug interaction software. J Am Pharm Assoc (Wash) 2001 Mar-Apr; 41 (2): 200-4.
7. Barrons R. Evaluation of personal digital assistant software for drug interactions. Am J Health Syst Pharm 2004 Feb 15; 61 (4): 380-5.
8. Perrin Y, Buclin T, Biollaz J. Drug interaction computer programs: which choice? [in French]. Schweiz Rundsch Med Prax 2004 Jun 2; 93 (23): 991-6.
9. Barla C, Mignot G, Chichmanian RM. Comparative study of data banks on drug interactions [in French]. Therapie 1992 Sep-Oct; 47 (5): 449-53.
10. WHO collaborating centre for drug statistics methodology, Norwegian Institute of Public Health, Oslo. WHO ATC/DDD applications [online]. Available from URL: http://www.whocc.no/atcddd/ [Accessed 2004 May-July].
11. Sweetman SC. Martindale - The complete drug reference. 33rd ed. London: The Pharmaceutical Press; 2002.
12. Hulley SB, Cummings SR, Browner WS. Designing clinical research: an epidemiologic approach. 2nd ed. Baltimore: Williams & Wilkins; 1998.
13. Stockley IH, editor. Stockley's drug interactions. 6th ed. London, Chicago: The Pharmaceutical Press; 2002.
14. Product Information: lithium carbonate. Columbus, OH: Roxane Laboratories Inc.; 2002.

15. Product Information: Euphylong(R), theophylline. Germany: Rote Liste; 2004.
16. Bjornsson TD, Callaghan JT, Einolf HJ, et al. The conduct of in vitro and in vivo drug-drug interaction studies: a PhRMA perspective. J Clin Pharmacol 2003 May; 43 (5): 443-69.
17. Hansten PD, Horn JR, Hazlet TK. ORCA: OpeRational ClassificAtion of drug interactions. J Am Pharm Assoc (Wash) 2001 Mar-Apr; 41 (2): 161-5.
18. Center for drug evaluation and research, U.S. food and drug administration. Electronic orange book [online]. Available from URL: http://www.fda.gov/cder/ob/default.htm [Accessed 2005 Aug 12].
19. Payne TH, Nichol WP, Hoey P, et al. Characteristics and override rates of order checks in a practitioner order entry system. Proc AMIA Symp 2002: 602-6.
20. Magnus D, Rodgers S, Avery AJ. GPs' views on computerized drug interaction alerts: questionnaire survey. J Clin Pharm Ther 2002 Oct; 27 (5): 377-82.
21. Weingart SN, Toth M, Sands DZ, et al. Physicians' decisions to override computerized drug alerts in primary care. Arch Intern Med 2003 Nov 24; 163 (21): 2625-31.
22. MacGregor FB, Abernethy VE, Dahabra S, et al. Hepatotoxicity of herbal remedies. Bmj 1989 Nov 4; 299 (6708): 1156-7.
23. Cavadas C, Araujo I, Cotrim MD, et al. In vitro study on the interaction of Valeriana officinalis L. extracts and their amino acids on GABAA receptor in rat brain. Arzneimittelforschung 1995 Jul; 45 (7): 753-5.
24. Miller LG. Herbal medicinals: selected clinical considerations focusing on known or potential drug-herb interactions. Arch Intern Med 1998 Nov 9; 158 (20): 2200-11.
25. Ortiz JG, Nieves-Natal J, Chavez P. Effects of Valeriana officinalis extracts on [3H]flunitrazepam binding, synaptosomal [3H]GABA uptake, and hippocampal [3H]GABA release. Neurochem Res 1999 Nov; 24 (11): 1373-8.
26. Ang-Lee MK, Moss J, Yuan CS. Herbal medicines and perioperative care. Jama 2001 Jul 11; 286 (2): 208-16.
27. Abebe W. Herbal medication: potential for adverse interactions with analgesic drugs. J Clin Pharm Ther 2002 Dec; 27 (6): 391-401.

28. Abebe W. An overview of herbal supplement utilization with particular emphasis on possible interactions with dental drugs and oral manifestations. J Dent Hyg 2003; 77 (1): 37-46.
29. Strandell J, Neil A, Carlin G. An approach to the in vitro evaluation of potential for cytochrome P450 enzyme inhibition from herbals and other natural remedies. Phytomedicine 2004 Feb; 11 (2-3): 98-104.
30. Lefebvre T, Foster BC, Drouin CE, et al. In vitro activity of commercial valerian root extracts against human cytochrome P450 3A4. J Pharm Pharm Sci 2004 Aug 12; 7 (2): 265-73.
31. Donovan JL, DeVane CL, Chavin KD, et al. Multiple night-time doses of valerian (Valeriana officinalis) had minimal effects on CYP3A4 activity and no effect on CYP2D6 activity in healthy volunteers. Drug Metab Dispos 2004 Dec; 32 (12): 1333-6.

# Prevalence of Drug-Drug Interactions at Hospital Entry, during Hospital Stay and at Hospital Discharge in a Department of Internal Medicine

Priska Vonbach[1], André Dubied[1], Stephan Krähenbühl[2], Jürg H Beer[3]

1 Hospital Pharmacy, Cantonal Hospital of Baden, Switzerland

2 Clinical Pharmacology & Toxicology, University Hospital Basel, Switzerland

3 Department of Medicine, Cantonal Hospital of Baden, Switzerland

**Abstract**

Introduction

The aim of this study was to assess potential drug-drug interactions (pDDIs) at hospital admission, during hospitalization and at discharge and to evaluate the number of pDDIs created during hospitalization due to changes in the medication. In addition, the clinical management of pDDIs by the physicians was investigated.

Methods

The medication of 851 patients was screened for pDDIs at hospital admission, during hospitalization and at discharge using the drug interaction screening program *Pharmavista*. Potential DDIs classified *major* and *moderate* were assessed separately. We focused in particular on four drug interaction groups to investigate the clinical management of pDDIs.

Results

At hospital discharge significantly more pDDIs per patient (1.6) were detected than at hospital admission (1.3) ($p = 0.005$). During hospitalization, the frequency of pDDIs was 2.5. When only *major* and *moderate* pDDIs per patient were considered, no significant difference between hospital admission and discharge was detected. The number of *major* or *moderate* pDDIs per drug pair administered was 4.5 at hospital admission, 1.6 during hospitalization and 2.3 at discharge. 47% of all *major* and *moderate* pDDIs at discharge were due to a medication change during hospitalization. Several deficiencies were detected regarding the management of clinically relevant pDDIs.

## Conclusion

Although the number of drugs increased from hospital admission to discharge by 50%, the number of *major* and *moderate* pDDIs per patient did not. In fact, the number of pDDI per drug pair administered was reduced by 50%. 47% of all *major* and *moderate* pDDIs at discharge were created by medication changes during hospitalization. Prescribing drugs with a low risk for pDDIs as well as careful monitoring for adverse drug reactions are important measures to prevent harm associated with pDDIs.

## Introduction

According to a recently published study one percent of all hospital admissions were caused by drug-drug interactions (DDIs), corresponding to 16% of all patients admitted with adverse drug reactions (ADR) [1]. In a recent review, an incidence of up to 2.8% of hospital admissions were found to be caused by ADRs due to DDIs [2]. The clinical outcome of a potential (p)DDI is often unknown, and epidemiological data dealing with this problem are rare. However, it was pointed out by Hamilton et al. [3] that exposure to DDIs was associated with a significantly increased risk of hospitalization.

The prevalence of pDDIs in the medication of ambulatory patients [4-6], of patients at hospital admission [7, 8], during hospitalization [9, 10], and at discharge [11-13] was assessed by numerous studies. One study assessed pDDIs for each patient at hospital admission, at discharge, and three months after discharge [14]. Changes in medication at the transition point from outpatient to inpatient care and back may increase the frequency of drug-related problems such as pDDIs [15, 16]. Drug modifications shortly before hospital discharge may be important in this context, because the monitoring of patients significantly declines after hospital discharge [17].

The aim of this study was to consecutively assess the frequency of pDDIs at hospital admission, during hospital stay on a medical ward and at hospital discharge. Further, we wanted to evaluate how many pDDIs were due to a change in prescriptions during hospitalization. Additionally, we attempted to analyze the clinical management of specific pDDIs by physicians.

## Methods

Study design, patients and data collection
The study was conducted at the Cantonal Hospital of Baden, Switzerland. The hospital is a 400-bed teaching institution serving a population of approximately 250'000 inhabitants.

Between February and July 2004, patients admitted consecutively to three medical wards were included in the study. Information on drugs prescribed at hospital admission, during hospital stay and at discharge was retrieved from clinical records and the hospital discharge letters. Medication prescribed "as required" was included, regardless of whether it was administered or not. The medication for inpatients was recorded on a specific day once a week and once per patient.

Demographic information (age and sex), length of hospital stay, main diagnosis (according to the international classification of diseases, $10^{th}$ revision (ICD-10)) and the number of additional diagnoses were obtained from the clinical records.

Classification of drug-drug interactions
The medication at hospital admission, during hospital stay and at hospital discharge was screened for pDDIs using the drug interaction screening program *Pharmavista* [18]. This drug interaction screening program originates from the "ABDA-Datenbank" published by the "Bundesvereinigung Deutscher Apothekerverbände" (federal organization of the German pharmacist associations). The program was chosen as a result of our evaluation of frequently used drug interaction screening programs [19]. In this publication, we recommended *Pharmavista* as the program with the highest sensitivity for detecting pDDIs, for its high negative and positive predictive values. For each interacting drug combination, *Pharmavista* provides information on the possible ADR, the clinical management and the mechanism of the DDI and provides literature references regarding the DDI.

The program classifies severities of DDIs into five categories: *major*[i], *moderate*[ii], *minor*[iii], *insignificant*[iv] and *unidentified source*[v]. In this study, DDIs of the severities *major*, *moderate* and *minor* were included for analysis; additionally, *major* and *moderate* DDIs were analyzed separately.

### Analysis of four groups of drug-drug interactions

We chose four well-known groups of DDIs to evaluate their prevalence and clinical management in more detail: drug-statin interactions, DDIs resulting in increased risk for hyperkalaemia, interactions between bisphosphonates and polyvalent cations and drug - nonsteroidal antiinflammatory drug (NSAID) interactions resulting in increased risk for gastrointestinal bleeding.

### Statistical analysis

Descriptive data were expressed as means with corresponding 95% confidence intervals (CIs), as medians and ranges, or as proportions. The Student's t-test was used for independent two-sample comparisons. A two-sided p-value less than 0.05 was considered statistically significant. Data were analyzed with R for Windows version 2.2.0 (R Development Core Team (2005), R Foundation for Statistical Computing, Vienna, Austria).

---

i *Major* interactions may be life-threatening, or intoxication or permanent damage may be induced. Normally, these drugs should not be administered together.

ii *Moderate* interactions frequently cause therapeutic difficulties, but the combinations may be administered if the patient is carefully monitored (laboratory parameters, for example quick value, or clinical symptoms).

iii *Minor* interactions may cause increased or reduced effects or interactions only concerning a certain subgroup (for example patients with renal or hepatic failure, slow acetylizers).

iv *Insignificant* interactions cause mainly no or unimportant effects and no special action is required.

v Within interactions classified as *unidentified source* no medical literature is available. Only isolated cases are cited or even postulated, and their clinical relevance is unclear.

## Results

### Patient characteristics and dropouts

A total of 851 patients were enrolled. The patient characteristics are displayed in Table I. The median age of the patients was 72 years. Slightly more than half of the patients were male (53%). Patients showed a median number of three coded diagnoses. However, due to the gain of economical importance of the coding, gaps were closed and the number of coded diagnoses increased to a median of four. Diseases of the circulatory system were most often specified as main diagnosis (27%).

Upon analysis of the prescriptions at hospital admission, 131 (15%) patients were excluded (115 patients because of insufficient information about medication and 16 patients because of incomplete medical history). Concerning the analysis of prescriptions at hospital discharge, 48 (5.6%) patients were excluded (43 patients died during hospitalization and five patients were excluded due to gaps in their medical history).

Table I: Characteristics of the 851 patients included in the study

| Characteristics | | n = 851 |
|---|---|---|
| Age - yr | Mean | 68.4 |
| | 95% Confidence interval | 67.4 - 69.4 |
| | Median | 72 |
| | Range | 18 - 99 |
| Sex - no. (%) | Male | 454 (53.3) |
| | Female | 397 (46.7) |
| Length of hospital stay - days | Mean | 12.0 |
| | 95% Confidence interval | 11.3 - 12.6 |
| | Median | 9 |
| | Range | 1 - 106 |
| Time between admission and collection of the drugs prescribed at the hospital stay[a] - days | Mean | 4.8 |
| | 95% Confidence interval | 4.5 - 5.0 |
| | Median | 4 |
| | Range | 0 - 34 |
| Coded number of diagnoses | Mean | 3.3 |
| | 95% Confidence interval | 3.2 - 3.4 |
| | Median | 3 |
| | Range | 1 - 9 |
| Main diagnoses (according to ICD-10) - no. (%) | Diseases of the circulatory system | 233 (27.4) |
| | Diseases of the digestive system | 99 (11.6) |
| | Diseases of the respiratory system | 88 (10.3) |
| | Neoplasms | 88 (10.3) |
| | Symptoms, signs and abnormal clinical and laboratory findings, not elsewhere classified | 82 (9.6) |
| | Diseases of the musculoskeletal system and connective tissue | 50 (5.9) |
| | Diseases of the nervous system | 39 (4.6) |
| | Factors influencing health status and contact with health services | 35 (4.1) |
| | Others (< 3%) | 137 (16.1) |

a. see Methods

ICD-10 = international classification of diseases, 10th revision, n = number of patients, no. = number, yr = year

## Prescribed drugs

The median total number of drugs prescribed was four at hospital admission, 11 during hospital stay and six at hospital discharge (Table II). During hospital stay, the median number of drugs without considering those prescribed "as required" was eight. The number of drugs prescribed at hospital discharge was significantly higher than at hospital admission ($p < 0.001$).

Table II: Number of drugs and number of drug pairs per patient at hospital admission, during hospitalization and at hospital discharge

|  |  | At hospital admission (n = 720) | During hospitalization (n = 851) | At hospital discharge (n = 803) |
|---|---|---|---|---|
| Number of drugs, excluding drugs prescribed "as required" | Mean | 4.1 | 7.8 | 6.2 |
|  | 95% CI | 3.9 - 4.4 | 7.5 - 8.1 | 6.0 - 6.4 |
|  | Median | 4 | 8 | 6 |
|  | Range | 0 - 17 | 0 - 27 | 0 - 19 |
| Number of drugs, prescribed "as required" | Mean | 0.2 | 3.7 | 0.4 |
|  | 95% CI | 0.2 - 0.3 | 3.6 - 3.9 | 0.4 - 0.5 |
|  | Median | 0 | 4 | 0 |
|  | Range | 0 - 4 | 0 - 10 | 0 - 6 |
| Total number of drugs | Mean | 4.3 | 11.6 | 6.6 |
|  | 95% CI | 4.1 - 4.6 | 11.2 - 11.9 | 6.4 - 6.9 |
|  | Median | 4 | 11 | 6 |
|  | Range | 0 - 17 | 2 - 34 | 0 - 21 |
| Number of drug pairs | Mean | 13.0 | 71.5 | 26.0 |
|  | 95% CI | 11.6 - 14.5 | 67.5 - 75.4 | 24.1 - 27.9 |
|  | Median | 6 | 55 | 15 |
|  | Range | 0 - 136 | 1 - 561 | 0 - 210 |

95% CI = 95% confidence interval, n = number of patients

Figure I displays the proportion of patients with at least one prescription belonging to the specified drug class (according to the anatomical therapeutical chemical (ATC) classification). Drugs affecting the central nervous system (e.g. oxazepam, lorazepam, valerian) were prescribed for 99% of the inpatients, but the majority of these drugs (68%) was prescribed "as required". At hospital admission, 44% of all patients were prescribed a drug affecting the central nervous system and 61% of the patients at hospital discharge. The other three most prevalent anatomical groups were drugs affecting the alimentary tract and metabolism (admission 46%, inpatients 79%, discharge 72%), drugs affecting the blood and blood forming organs (admission 45%, inpatients 80%, discharge 60%) and drugs affecting the cardiovascular system (admission 61%, inpatients 77%, discharge 71%). These four groups represented 82% of all drugs at hospital admission, 84% during hospital stay and 85% at hospital discharge.

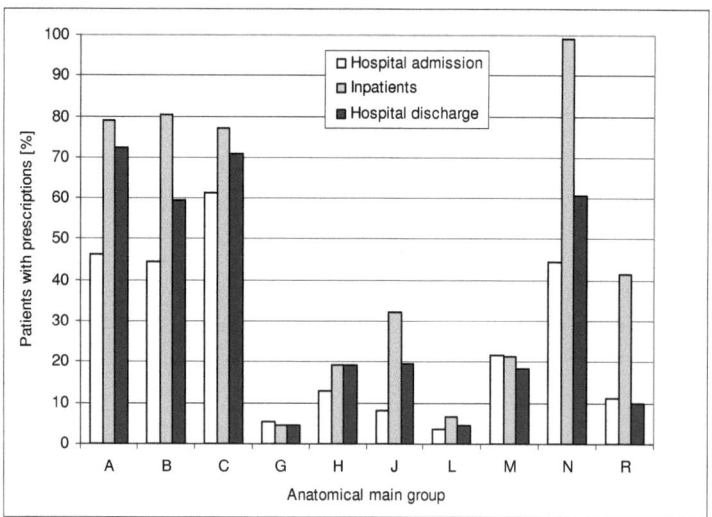

Figure I: Proportion of patients (> 5%) with prescriptions belonging to the drug classes according to the anatomical therapeutical chemical (ATC) classification at hospital admission (n = 720), inpatients (n = 851) and hospital discharge (n = 803)

n = number of patients; anatomical main groups: A = alimentary tract and metabolism, B = blood and blood forming organs, C = cardiovascular system, D = genito urinary system and sex hormones, H = systemic hormonal preparations, exclusive sex hormones and insulins, J = antiinfectives for systemic use, L = antineoplastic and immunomodulating agent, M = musculo-skeletal system, N = nervous system, R = respiratory system

During hospital stay, all drug classes – except drugs affecting the genito-urinary system and drugs affecting the musculo-skeletal system – had the highest prescription frequency. Antiinfectives for systemic use as well as drugs affecting the respiratory system were administered to four times more patients during hospitalization as compared to patients at hospital admission or discharge.

Drug-drug interactions in general

The prevalence of pDDIs at hospital admission, during hospital stay as well as at hospital discharge is shown in detail in Table III. At hospital entry 47% of the patients had at least one pDDI. This figure increased during hospitalization to 73% and dropped at discharge to 59%. Considering pDDI classified as *major* or *moderate* only, the frequencies were 30% at hospital entry, 56% during hospitalization and 31% at discharge. When expressed per patient, the corresponding figures for *major* and *moderate* pDDIs were 0.59 at entry, 1.11 during hospitalization and 0.60 at discharge. Regarding *major* and *moderate* pDDIs expressed per patient, the value for inpatients was significantly higher than at admission or at discharge, whereas there was no difference between entry and discharge.

Table III: Prevalence of potential drug-drug interactions (pDDIs) in the medication at hospital admission, during hospitalization and at hospital discharge

|  |  | At hospital admission (n = 720) | During hospitalization (n = 851) | At hospital discharge (n = 803) |
|---|---|---|---|---|
| Number of patients with ≥ one *major* pDDI | no. (%) | 4 (0.6) | 26 (3.1) | 5 (0.6) |
|  | 95% CI (%) | 0.0 - 1.2 | 1.8 - 4.0 | 0.0 - 1.2 |
| Number of patients with ≥ one *major* or *moderate* pDDI | no. (%) | 215 (29.9) | 478 (56.2) | 248 (30.9) |
|  | 95% CI (%) | 26.5 - 33.3 | 52.8 - 59.6 | 27.6 - 34.2 |
| Number of patients with ≥ one *major*, *moderate* or *minor* pDDI | no. (%) | 339 (47.1) | 625 (73.4) | 473 (58.9) |
|  | 95% CI (%) | 43.4 - 50.8 | 70.4 - 76.4 | 55.4 - 62.4 |
| Number of *major* pDDIs per patient | Mean | 0.01 | 0.03 | 0.01 |
|  | 95% CI | 0.00 - 0.01 | 0.02 - 0.05 | 0.00 - 0.01 |
|  | Median | 0 | 0 | 0 |
|  | Range | 0 - 1 | 0 - 2 | 0 - 1 |
| Number of *major* or *moderate* pDDIs per patient | Mean | 0.59 | 1.11 | 0.60 |
|  | 95% CI | 0.50 - 0.68 | 1.00 - 1.21 | 0.51 - 0.68 |
|  | Median | 0 | 1 | 0 |
|  | Range | 0 - 12 | 0 - 11 | 0 - 9 |
| Number of *major*, *moderate* or *minor* pDDIs per patient | Mean | 1.3 | 2.5 | 1.6 |
|  | 95% CI | 1.1 - 1.4 | 2.3 - 2.7 | 1.4 - 1.7 |
|  | Median | 0 | 1 | 1 |
|  | Range | 0 - 16 | 0 - 19 | 0 - 18 |

95% CI = 95% confidence interval, n = number of patients, no. = number

The prevalence of *major* or *moderate* pDDIs in proportion to the number of drugs (Table IV) declines from 13.7% (0.59 of 4.3) at hospital admission to 9.6% (1.11 of 11.6) during hospitalization and to 9.1% (0.60 of 6.6) at discharge. The ratio between the number of *major* and *moderate* pDDIs and the number of drug pairs was lowest during hospitalization (1.6%, 1.11 of 71.5) and highest at hospital admission (4.5%, 0.59 of 13.0).

Table IV: Prevalence of *major* or *moderate* potential drug-drug interactions (pDDIs) in proportion to the number of drugs and to the number of drug pairs at hospital admission, during hospitalization and at hospital discharge

|  |  | At hospital admission (n = 720) | During hospitalization (n = 851) | At hospital discharge (n = 803) |
|---|---|---|---|---|
| Total number of drugs | Mean | 4.3 | 11.6 | 6.6 |
| Number of *major* or *moderate* pDDIs per patient | Mean | 0.59 | 1.11 | 0.60 |
| Number of drug pairs | Mean | 13.0 | 71.5 | 26.0 |
| Mean number of *major* or *moderate* pDDI / mean number of drugs | Ratio (%) | 13.7 | 9.6 | 9.1 |
| Mean number of *major* or *moderate* pDDI / mean number of drug pairs | Ratio (%) | 4.5 | 1.6 | 2.3 |

n = number of patients

For 697 patients, all prescriptions at admission, during hospital stay and at discharge could be analyzed. Focusing on *major* and *moderate* pDDIs, 406 were present at hospital admission, whereof 103 (25%) were eliminated during the first days of hospitalization. During hospitalization, an additional 450 pDDIs were generated due to new medications, resulting in a total of 753 pDDIs. Almost half of these pDDIs (365, 49%) were eliminated at hospital discharge, when only eight new pDDIs were detected compared to the inpatient medication. Out of 396 DDIs at hospital discharge, 185 (47%) were due to a medication change during the hospital stay. Regarding *major* pDDIs only, out of three pDDIs at hospital admission two were eliminated during hospitalization. During hospital stay, 21 *major* pDDIs were created, whereof 18 were eliminated at hospital discharge.

Table V lists all *major* pDDIs and the most prevalent *moderate* pDDIs, which account for 62% of all *major* and *moderate* pDDIs at hospital admission, for 67% at hospital stay and for 61% at hospital discharge.

Table V: *Major* and *moderate* potential drug-drug interactions (pDDIs) at hospital admission, during hospitalization and at hospital discharge. All *major* pDDIs are listed, whereas for the *moderate* pDDIs only those are listed with a frequency of ≥ 3% among the patients.

| Drug combination | Potential adverse effect | Severity | Patients with pDDIs - no. (%) | | |
|---|---|---|---|---|---|
| | | | At hospital admission (n = 720) | During hospitalization (n = 851) | At hospital discharge (n = 803) |
| Potassium + potassium-sparing diuretic | Hyperkalaemia | Major | 1 (0.1) | 12 (1.4) | 3 (0.4) |
| Beta-sympathomimetic agent + non-cardio-selective beta-blocker | Decreased effect of beta-sympathomimetic agent | Major | 2 (0.3) | 6 (0.7) | 0 (0.0) |
| Macrolide antibiotic + statin | Increased risk of myopathy including rhabdomyolysis | Major | 0 (0.0) | 4 (0.5) | 1 (0.1) |
| Heparinoid + salicylate (high-dose) | Increased risk of bleeding | Major | 0 (0.0) | 4 (0.5) | 0 (0.0) |
| MAO inhibitor + opioid | Increased risk of adverse reactions affecting the central nervous system | Major | 1 (0.1) | 1 (0.1) | 1 (0.1) |
| Heparinoids + salicylate (low-dose) | Increased risk of bleeding | Moderate | 6 (0.8) | 193 (22.7) | 31 (3.9) |
| Diuretic + glucocorticoid | Risk for hypokalaemia | Moderate | 65 (9.0) | 106 (12.5) | 67 (8.3) |
| Diuretic + NSAID | Decreased diuretic and antihypertensive effect | Moderate | 40 (5.6) | 38 (4.5) | 28 (3.5) |
| ACE inhibitor + NSAID | Decreased antihypertensive effect | Moderate | 22 (3.1) | 36 (4.2) | 20 (2.5) |
| Glucocorticoid + NSAID | Increased risk of bleeding | Moderate | 24 (3.3) | 35 (4.1) | 22 (2.7) |
| Beta-blocker + insulin | Increased risk for hypoglycaemia | Moderate | 12 (1.7) | 35 (4.1) | 20 (2.5) |
| ACE inhibitor + potassium salt | Risk for hyperkalaemia | Moderate | 5 (0.7) | 34 (4.0) | 7 (0.9) |
| ACE inhibitor + potassium-sparing diuretic | Risk for hyperkalaemia | Moderate | 22 (3.1) | 30 (3.5) | 25 (3.1) |
| Antidiabetes agent + glucocorticoid | Impaired blood glucose control | Moderate | 11 (1.5) | 23 (2.7) | 19 (2.4) |
| Beta-blocker + NSAID | Decreased antihypertensive effect | Moderate | 21 (2.9) | 22 (2.6) | 16 (2.0) |
| Bisphosphonate + polyvalent cation | Decreased bioavailability of bisphosphonate | Moderate | 18 (2.5) | 19 (2.2) | 14 (1.7) |
| Oral anticoagulant + thyroid hormone | Decreased anticoagulant effectiveness | Moderate | 10 (1.4) | 10 (1.2) | 15 (1.9) |

ACE = angiotensin-converting enzyme, MAO = monoamine oxidase, n = number of patients, no. = number, NSAID = nonsteroidal antiinflammatory drug

More than 70% of all *major* and *moderate* pDDIs are caused by a pharmacodynamic mechanism (hospital admission 71%, inpatients 76%, hospital discharge 72%), whereas pharmacokinetic mechanisms were observed in 27% of pDDIs at hospital admission, in 22% of pDDIs during hospital stay and in 26% of pDDIs at hospital discharge. The remaining pDDIs had a combined or an unknown mechanism. Concerning the pharmacokinetic pDDIs, approximately half of them could be explained by inhibition of induction of metabolic enzymes, in particular the cytochrome P450 (CYP) system (15% of pDDIs at hospital admission and at hospital discharge, 12% at hospitalization).

Drug - statin interactions at hospital discharge
At hospital discharge, nine drug - statin interactions resulting in an increased risk for myopathy and rhabdomyolysis were observed. Six pDDIs were due to atorvastatin, two to simvastatin and one to pravastatin. As CYP3A4-inhibiting drugs amiodarone (4), verapamil (2) and clarithromycin (1) were found. Within two statin - cyclosporine interactions (atorvastatin and pravastatin) inhibition of the organic anion transporting polypeptide (OATP-2) mediated hepatic uptake of statins by cyclosporine, leading to increased statin plasma concentrations, is supposed [20, 21]. Five drug - statin interactions resulted from new prescriptions (atorvastatin in a patient treated with cyclosporine, atorvastatin in two patients treated with amiodarone, simvastatin in a patient treated with verapamil, and clarithromycin in a patient treated with atorvastatin).

Potential drug-drug interactions resulting in increased risk for hyperkalaemia
At hospital discharge, 37 pDDIs (in 36 patients) resulting in an increased risk for hyperkalaemia were detected, whereof 25 (68%) were attributed to the combination angiotensin-converting enzyme (ACE) inhibitors and potassium-sparing diuretics. Three (8%) of these pDDIs (potassium salts and potassium-sparing diuretics) were classified as *major*. A potassium-wasting diuretic (loop diuretic and/or thiazide) was included in the medication regimen of 31 (84%) of these patients. The mean serum potassium level at discharge was 4.0 mmol/L (95% CI 3.8 - 4.1 mmol/L, range 2.9 - 5.2 mmol/L). The mean estimated creatinine clearance was 66 mL/min (95% CI 53 - 79 mL/min, range 16 - 161 mL/min). Two patients with the combination of an ACE inhibitor with spironolactone showed potassium levels above the normal range

(3.5 - 4.8 mmol/L). One of these patients (serum potassium level 5.2 mmol/L) had a severely impaired renal function (estimated creatinine clearance 16 mL/min), which represents an additional risk factor for hyperkalaemia. The other patient (serum potassium level 4.9 mmol/L) had only a slight impairment of renal function (estimated creatinine clearance 64 mL/min) and was treated with a loop diuretic.

Interactions between bisphosphonates and polyvalent cations at hospital discharge
67% of the patients treated with a bisphosphonate (14 of 21 patients, 13 alendronic acid, 1 clodronic acid) were discharged with a polyvalent cation (13 calcium carbonate, 1 magnesium aspartate). According to the hospital discharge letters, in 12 patients the polyvalent cation was to be administered with an insufficient time interval to the bisphosphonate. Only two patients were advised to take the calcium at lunchtime.

Drug - nonsteroidal antiinflammatory drug interactions resulting in increased risk for gastrointestinal bleeding
Drug - NSAID interactions resulting in increased risk for gastrointestinal bleeding (NSAIDs combined with oral anticoagulants, glucocorticoids or thrombocyte aggregation inhibitors) rose from 5.3% (38 of 720 patients) at hospital admission to 8.3% (67 of 803 patients) at hospital discharge. At hospital discharge, 5.5% (44) of all patients received the combination of a NSAID and a thrombocyte aggregation inhibitor (at admission 1.4%), 2.7% (22) were treated with the combination NSAID and glucocorticoid (at admission 3.3%) and one patient (0.1%) was prescribed an oral anticoagulant and a NSAID (at admission 0.6%). 42 of the 44 thrombocyte aggregation inhibitor - NSAID interactions were due to the combination with clopidogrel and/or low-dose aspirin. Approximately half of these patients (20) were treated with an antacid drug such as a proton pump inhibitor (PPI) in addition. One patient was treated with the combination low-dose aspirin and ibuprofen, which can blunt the effect of aspirin when ingested together [22].

## Discussion

Our study shows that the number of drugs prescribed per patient increased significantly from hospital admission to discharge, whereas the number of *major* and *moderate* pDDIs per patient was not higher at discharge compared to admission. During hospitalization, the number of prescribed drugs as well as the number of *major* and *moderate* pDDIs per patient was significantly higher than at hospital admission and discharge. In relation to the number of drugs as well as to the number of drug pairs, the prevalence of pDDIs even decreased from hospital entry to discharge. Approximately 50% of all *moderate* and *major* pDDI at discharge were due to changes in the medication during hospitalization.

The figures found in our study compare well with similar reports in the literature. Egger et al. retrospectively screened the medication for pDDIs of 500 medical patients only at hospital admission and discharge, but not at hospital stay [12]. The patient characteristics as well as the drugs used were quite similar to those in our study. The results showed that – although another drug interaction screening program (Drug-Reax [23]) was used – the prevalence of patients with at least one pDDI at hospital admission (48%) and at hospital discharge (60%) was comparable to our results. Straubhaar et al. studied the prevalence of pDDIs in patients with heart failure. They found that 68% of patients at hospital admission and 89% of patients at hospital discharge had at least one pDDI [13]. These data are not directly comparable with our study because of different patient characteristics and drug prescriptions. Köhler et al. used the same data base ("ABDA Datenbank") as *Pharmavista* for screening prescriptions of patients at hospital entry and discharge [14]. Unfortunately, the classification of severities by *Pharmavista* changed between 1996 and 2004, and therefore the results are not directly comparable. The mean number of all pDDIs per patient at hospital admission and discharge were 1.5 (vs 1.4 in our study) and 1.7 (vs 1.8), respectively. The proportion of patients free of pDDIs at hospital admission was 44% (vs 53% in our study), and 40% at discharge (vs 41%). Concerning *major* pDDIs, Köhler et al. found a slight increase in the number of pDDIs per patient between hospital admission and hospital discharge (0.02 at admission, 0.04 at discharge), which is in contrast with the results of our study.

Potential DDIs with a higher frequency during hospitalization were potassium supplements in patients treated with potassium sparing diuretics or ACE inhibitors or angiotensin receptor blockers, macrolide antibiotics in patients treated with statins, non-cardioselective beta-blockers in patients treated with $\beta_2$-sympathomimetics, beta-blockers in diabetics and the combination of heparinoids in patients treated with cardiovascular or analgesic doses of aspirin.

Regarding the combination of potassium supplements with potassium sparing diuretics, ACE inhibitors or angiotensin receptor blockers, this combination appears to be acceptable in the hospital, since serum potassium levels and renal function can be monitored closely. However, when patients are discharged, the combination should be discontinued in order to avoid potentially life-threatening hyperkalaemia. In our study, 4.5% (36 patients) of the patients at hospital discharge were exposed to pDDIs that could have resulted in hyperkalaemia. All of these patients had the combination spironolactone and ACE inhibitor, which is common in patients with heart failure [6, 13]. None of the patients was discharged with potassium supplements in combination with spironolactone, ACE inhibitors or angiotensin receptor blockers.

The combination of macrolides (erythromycin, roxithromycin, clarithromycin) with statins metabolized by CYP3A4 (atorvastatin, lovastatin, simvastatin) should be avoided, since it increases the risk for myopathies [24, 25]. The risk for rhabdomyolysis in patients treated with a statin without pDDI has been estimated to be in the range of 1:10'000 patient years [26]. This risk increases approximately by a factor of ten (to 1:1'000 patient years), when a CYP3A4 inhibitor is co-administered [6]. In the case of macrolide antibiotics, which are usually used for one to two weeks only, the statin should be stopped during treatment. In our patients, the prevalence of drug - statin interactions in statin-treated patients declined from 8.4% (10 pDDIs in 119 statin-treated patients) at hospital admission to 5.6% (12 pDDIs in 213 statin-treated patients) during hospital stay and 4.0% (9 pDDIs in 226 statin-treated patients) at hospital discharge. Rätz et al. found a prevalence of 6.9% drug - statin interactions in ambulatory patients with statin treatment [6]. Out of nine drug - statin interactions at hospital discharge, seven could have been avoided by choosing a statin which is not metabolized by CYP3A4 [27].

The concomitant use of non-cardioselective beta-blockers with $\beta_2$-symapthomimetics should generally be avoided. Non-cardioselective beta-blockers not only decrease the efficacy of $\beta_2$-sympathomimetics, but are also mostly contraindicated in the patients where $\beta_2$-sympathomimetics are indicated. If beta-blockers are to be used in such patients, cardioselective beta-blockers should be preferred but only under close monitoring of pulmonary function [28].

The use of beta-blockers in patients with diabetes mellitus is a matter of debate. Due to the possibility that the symptoms associated with hypoglycaemia are mitigated and glycogenolysis is impaired, the risk for hypoglycaemia may be increased. While this is the case for non-cardioselective beta-blockers [29], cardioselective beta-blockers can be considered to be safe in diabetics [30, 31]. We therefore advise to avoid non-cardioselective beta-blockers in diabetics and to prefer cardioselective beta-blockers, but only in patients with a clear indication. Furthermore, the patients should know that tachycardia may not develop despite hypoglycaemia, but that sweating may be increased [30].

The combination of thrombocyte aggregation inhibitors with heparins is associated with a higher risk of bleeding than either treatment alone, but this risk is outweighed by the improved antithrombotic efficacy of this combination in certain groups of patients such as patients with an acute coronary syndrome [32, 33]. On the other hand, analgesic doses of aspirin or other NSAIDs should most probably not be combined with heparins, due to the local effects of NSAIDs in the gastrointestinal tract, which may bleed. While the combination of NSAIDs with oral anticoagulation has clearly been shown to be associated with a very high risk for bleeding and should therefore be avoided [34], such data do – to the best of our knowledge – not exist for the combination with heparin.

Limitations

Concerning the medication at hospital admission, possibly incomplete medical record documentation has to be considered. Recent studies showed discrepancies in 40 to 50% of patients between medical record and patient-reported use of drugs [35-37]. For non-prescription NSAIDs, disagreement was found in 74% of patients' medication [37]. A systematic review found that up to 61% of cases had at least one omission error in prescription medication histories [38].

Another limitation concerns drugs prescribed "as required", since we do not know if patients actually ingested this medication. However, DDIs might have occurred if they had been administered to the patient. Therefore, physicians should be careful regarding pDDIs when prescribing drugs "as required".

Further, clinically manifest DDIs were not a concern of this study and therefore we use the expression *potential* DDI. Data about negative clinical outcomes caused by DDIs are rare, but some retrospective studies have been published. Ray et al. showed that the rate of sudden death from cardiac causes was five times as high among patients who concurrently used CYP3A inhibitors and erythromycin [39]. Juurlink et al. calculated odds ratios of 6.6 for hypoglycaemia in patients treated with glyburide in combination with co-trimoxazole, 11.7 for digoxin toxicity in patients treated with clarithromycin and 20.3 for hyperkalaemia in patients with ACE inhibitors combined with potassium-sparing diuretics [40].

Another limitation concerns the drug interaction screening program. Although our evaluation showed that *Pharmavista* provides high sensitivity and sophisticated information about DDIs (mechanism and clinical management) [19], some improvement is desirable. For example, pulmonary inhalation of glucocorticoids is not distinguished from systemic use of glucocorticoids, and thus the combination of inhaled glucocorticoid and low-dose aspirin is designated as a *moderate* pDDI. The same problem is present with diuretic drugs and pulmonary glucocorticoid treatment. No information about negative outcomes concerning these combinations with locally administered glucocorticoids was found in *Stockley's drug interactions* [41], a comprehensive monograph of DDIs. Furthermore, no differentiation is made between cardioselective and non-cardioselective beta-blocking agents concerning use in diabetics.

## Conclusion

Although the number of drugs increased from hospital admission to discharge by 50%, the number of *major* and *moderate* pDDIs per patient did not increase. Despite of these results, it is important to realize that 47% of all *major* and *moderate* pDDIs at discharge were created by medication changes during hospitalization. Prescribing drugs with a low risk for pDDIs as well as careful monitoring for ADRs are important measures to prevent harm associated with pDDIs.

## References

1. Pirmohamed M, James S, Meakin S, et al. Adverse drug reactions as cause of admission to hospital: prospective analysis of 18 820 patients. Bmj 2004 Jul 3; 329 (7456): 15-9.
2. Jankel CA, Fitterman LK. Epidemiology of drug-drug interactions as a cause of hospital admissions. Drug Saf 1993 Jul; 9 (1): 51-9.
3. Hamilton RA, Briceland LL, Andritz MH. Frequency of hospitalization after exposure to known drug-drug interactions in a Medicaid population. Pharmacotherapy 1998 Sep-Oct; 18 (5): 1112-20.
4. Mitchell GW, Stanaszek WF, Nichols NB. Documenting drug-drug interactions in ambulatory patients. Am J Hosp Pharm 1979 May; 36 (5): 653-7.
5. Costa AJ. Potential drug interactions in an ambulatory geriatric population. Fam Pract 1991 Sep; 8 (3): 234-6.
6. Ratz Bravo AE, Tchambaz L, Krahenbuhl-Melcher A, et al. Prevalence of potentially severe drug-drug interactions in ambulatory patients with dyslipidaemia receiving HMG-CoA reductase inhibitor therapy. Drug Saf 2005; 28 (3): 263-75.
7. Gosney M, Tallis R. Prescription of contraindicated and interacting drugs in elderly patients admitted to hospital. Lancet 1984 Sep 8; 2 (8402): 564-7.
8. Manchon ND, Bercoff E, Lemarchand P, et al. [Incidence and severity of drug interactions in the elderly: a prospective study of 639 patients]. Rev Med Interne 1989 Nov-Dec; 10 (6): 521-5.
9. Gronroos PE, Irjala KM, Huupponen RK, et al. A medication database - a tool for detecting drug interactions in hospital. Eur J Clin Pharmacol 1997; 53 (1): 13-7.
10. Wiltink EH. Medication control in hospitals: a practical approach to the problem of drug-drug interactions. Pharm World Sci 1998 Aug; 20 (4): 173-7.
11. Bonetti PO, Hartmann K, Kuhn M, et al. [Potential drug interactions and number of prescription drugs with special instructions at hospital discharge]. Schweiz Rundsch Med Prax 2000 Jan 27; 89 (5): 182-9.
12. Egger SS, Drewe J, Schlienger RG. Potential drug-drug interactions in the medication of medical patients at hospital discharge. Eur J Clin Pharmacol 2003 Mar; 58 (11): 773-8.

13. Straubhaar B, Krahenbuhl S, Schlienger RG. The prevalence of potential drug-drug interactions in patients with heart failure at hospital discharge. Drug Saf 2006; 29 (1): 79-90.
14. Kohler GI, Bode-Boger SM, Busse R, et al. Drug-drug interactions in medical patients: effects of in-hospital treatment and relation to multiple drug use. Int J Clin Pharmacol Ther 2000 Nov; 38 (11): 504-13.
15. Himmel W, Tabache M, Kochen MM. What happens to long-term medication when general practice patients are referred to hospital? Eur J Clin Pharmacol 1996; 50 (4): 253-7.
16. Smith L, McGowan L, Moss-Barclay C, et al. An investigation of hospital generated pharmaceutical care when patients are discharged home from hospital. Br J Clin Pharmacol 1997 Aug; 44 (2): 163-5.
17. Cook RI, Render M, Woods DD. Gaps in the continuity of care and progress on patient safety. Bmj 2000 Mar 18; 320 (7237): 791-4.
18. e-mediat. Pharmavista - information for healthcare professionals. Version February 2005. e-mediat AG, Schönbühl, Switzerland; 2005.
19. Vonbach P, Dubied A, Krahenbuhl S, et al. Evaluation of drug interaction screening programs. Forum Med Suisse 2005; 8 S (Suppl 23): P15.
20. Hsiang B, Zhu Y, Wang Z, et al. A novel human hepatic organic anion transporting polypeptide (OATP2). Identification of a liver-specific human organic anion transporting polypeptide and identification of rat and human hydroxymethylglutaryl-CoA reductase inhibitor transporters. J Biol Chem 1999 Dec 24; 274 (52): 37161-8.
21. Shitara Y, Itoh T, Sato H, et al. Inhibition of transporter-mediated hepatic uptake as a mechanism for drug-drug interaction between cerivastatin and cyclosporin A. J Pharmacol Exp Ther 2003 Feb; 304 (2): 610-6.
22. Catella-Lawson F, Reilly MP, Kapoor SC, et al. Cyclooxygenase inhibitors and the antiplatelet effects of aspirin. N Engl J Med 2001 Dec 20; 345 (25): 1809-17.
23. Klasco RK. DRUG-REAX System. Vol. 113. Thomson MICROMEDEX, Greenwood Village, Colorado; 2002.
24. Omar MA, Wilson JP. FDA adverse event reports on statin-associated rhabdomyolysis. Ann Pharmacother 2002 Feb; 36 (2): 288-95.

25. Roten L, Schoenenberger RA, Krahenbuhl S, et al. Rhabdomyolysis in association with simvastatin and amiodarone. Ann Pharmacother 2004 Jun; 38 (6): 978-81.
26. Silverstein FE, Graham DY, Senior JR, et al. Misoprostol reduces serious gastrointestinal complications in patients with rheumatoid arthritis receiving nonsteroidal anti-inflammatory drugs. A randomized, double-blind, placebo-controlled trial. Ann Intern Med 1995 Aug 15; 123 (4): 241-9.
27. Bellosta S, Paoletti R, Corsini A. Safety of statins: focus on clinical pharmacokinetics and drug interactions. Circulation 2004 Jun 15; 109 (23 Suppl 1): III50-7.
28. Salpeter SR, Ormiston TM, Salpeter EE. Cardioselective beta-blockers in patients with reactive airway disease: a meta-analysis. Ann Intern Med 2002 Nov 5; 137 (9): 715-25.
29. Lager I, Blohme G, Smith U. Effect of cardioselective and non-selective beta-blockade on the hypoglycaemic response in insulin-dependent diabetics. Lancet 1979 Mar 3; 1 (8114): 458-62.
30. Sawicki PT, Siebenhofer A. Betablocker treatment in diabetes mellitus. J Intern Med 2001 Jul; 250 (1): 11-7.
31. Deedwania PC, Giles TD, Klibaner M, et al. Efficacy, safety and tolerability of metoprolol CR/XL in patients with diabetes and chronic heart failure: experiences from MERIT-HF. Am Heart J 2005 Jan; 149 (1): 159-67.
32. ISIS. ISIS-3: a randomised comparison of streptokinase vs tissue plasminogen activator vs anistreplase and of aspirin plus heparin vs aspirin alone among 41,299 cases of suspected acute myocardial infarction. ISIS-3 (Third International Study of Infarct Survival) Collaborative Group. Lancet 1992 Mar 28; 339 (8796): 753-70.
33. GUSTO. An international randomized trial comparing four thrombolytic strategies for acute myocardial infarction. The GUSTO investigators. N Engl J Med 1993 Sep 2; 329 (10): 673-82.
34. Knijff-Dutmer EA, Schut GA, van de Laar MA. Concomitant coumarin-NSAID therapy and risk for bleeding. Ann Pharmacother 2003 Jan; 37 (1): 12-6.
35. Lau HS, Florax C, Porsius AJ, et al. The completeness of medication histories in hospital medical records of patients admitted to general internal medicine wards. Br J Clin Pharmacol 2000 Jun; 49 (6): 597-603.

36. Cornish PL, Knowles SR, Marchesano R, et al. Unintended medication discrepancies at the time of hospital admission. Arch Intern Med 2005 Feb 28; 165 (4): 424-9.
37. Abdolrasulnia M, Weichold N, Shewchuk R, et al. Agreement between medical record documentation and patient-reported use of nonsteroidal anti-inflammatory drugs. Am J Health Syst Pharm 2006 Apr 15; 63 (8): 744-7.
38. Tam VC, Knowles SR, Cornish PL, et al. Frequency, type and clinical importance of medication history errors at admission to hospital: a systematic review. Cmaj 2005 Aug 30; 173 (5): 510-5.
39. Ray WA, Murray KT, Meredith S, et al. Oral erythromycin and the risk of sudden death from cardiac causes. N Engl J Med 2004 Sep 9; 351 (11): 1089-96.
40. Juurlink DN, Mamdani M, Kopp A, et al. Drug-drug interactions among elderly patients hospitalized for drug toxicity. Jama 2003 Apr 2; 289 (13): 1652-8.
41. Stockley IH, editor. Stockley's drug interactions. 6th ed. London, Chicago: The Pharmaceutical Press; 2002.

# Clinical Pharmacist's Intervention to improve the Management of potential Drug-Drug Interactions in a Department of Internal Medicine

Priska Vonbach[1], André Dubied[1], Jürg H Beer[2], Stephan Krähenbühl[3]

1 Hospital Pharmacy, Cantonal Hospital of Baden, Switzerland

2 Department of Medicine, Cantonal Hospital of Baden, Switzerland

3 Clinical Pharmacology & Toxicology, University Hospital Basel, Switzerland

**Abstract**

Introduction
The aim of this study was to improve the clinical management of potential drug-drug interactions (pDDIs) by pharmacist interventions during hospitalization and at hospital discharge.

Methods
During the first study period inpatients in three medical wards and during the second study period patients discharged from three medical wards were screened for *major* and *moderate* pDDIs using the drug interaction screening program *Pharmavista*. After assessment for clinical relevance of the detected pDDIs by a pharmacist, written recommendations and information about the pDDIs were sent to the physicians. Feedback from the physicians and their subsequent implementations were analyzed.

Results
During the first study period, 502 inpatients were exposed to 567 *major* or *moderate* pDDIs. 419 (74%) of these pDDIs were judged clinically relevant by the pharmacist. 349 recommendations including pDDI information, and 70 simply information leaflets were handed out to the physicians. 80% (278 of 349) of the recommendations were accepted. At hospital discharge, in 78% (47 of 60 reviewed instances, which were accepted) the drug changes due to the recommendations were implemented.

During the second study period, 792 patients at hospital discharge were exposed to 392 *major* and *moderate* pDDIs. 258 (66%) pDDIs were assessed as clinically relevant by the pharmacist. 247 recommendations including pDDI information, and 11 simply information leaflets were sent to the physicians. 73% (180 of 247) of the recommendations were accepted. One year after hospital discharge, 11 of 13 drug changes due to recommendations were still existent.

Overall, in 50% and 46%, respectively, of all *major* and *moderate* pDDIs detected by *Pharmavista,* clinical management was adapted accordingly.

## Conclusion

The management of clinically relevant pDDIs can be improved by physicians' advice of clinical pharmacists. Changes in medication due to pDDIs were found to persist up to one year after hospital discharge.

## Introduction

Medication errors, adverse drug events (ADEs) and adverse drug reactions (ADRs) are common and clinically important problems. ADEs and ADRs are associated with considerable morbidity and mortality [1-12]. According to a recently published study one percent of all hospital admissions was caused by drug-drug interactions (DDIs), corresponding to 16% of all patients admitted with ADRs [9]. A review of nine ADR studies found an incidence up to 2.8% of DDIs as a cause of hospital admissions [13]. In recent years major progress in our understanding of DDIs has been made, particularly in the molecular mechanism by which drugs interact. But our ability to appropriately apply this information to specific patients has lagged behind and patients continue to suffer from adverse DDIs.

Changes in medication at the transition point from outpatient to inpatient care and vice versa may increase the frequency of drug-related problems such as potential (p)DDIs [10, 14-16]. In our study on the prevalence of pDDIs during hospital stay, 47% of all pDDIs at discharge were created by medication changes during hospitalization. Furthermore, several deficiencies were detected regarding the clinical management of pDDIs.

The aim of this study was to improve the clinical management of pDDIs by pharmacist interventions during hospitalization and at hospital discharge.

## Methods

Patients and data collection

The intervention study was conducted at the Cantonal Hospital of Baden, Switzerland. The hospital is a 400-bed teaching institution serving a population of approximately 250'000 inhabitants. The Clinic of Medicine is not (yet) equipped with a computerized physician order entry (CPOE) and therefore no automatic DDI order check was available.

Between February and May 2005, patients admitted to three medical wards were included in the first part of the study (intervention period during hospitalization). Information on drugs prescribed during hospitalization was retrieved from clinical records and was collected on a fixed day once a week and once per patient.

Between June and October 2005, patients discharged from three medical wards were included in the second part of the study (intervention period at hospital discharge). Information on drugs prescribed at discharge was obtained from the hospital discharge letters on the day of discharge.

Demographic information (age and sex), length of hospital stay, main diagnosis (according to the international classification of diseases, 10$^{th}$ revision (ICD-10)) and the number of additional diagnoses were obtained from the clinical records.

Classification of the potential drug-drug interactions

Medication was screened for pDDIs using the drug interaction screening program *Pharmavista* [17]. This drug interaction screening program originates from the "ABDA-Datenbank" published by the "Bundesvereinigung Deutscher Apotheker-verbände" (federal organization of the German pharmacist associations). The program was chosen as a result of our evaluation of nine drug interaction screening programs [18]. In this publication, we recommended *Pharmavista* as the program with the highest sensitivity for detecting pDDIs, despite the limitation that it is written in German. The program classifies severities of DDIs into five categories: *major*[i], *moderate*[ii], *minor*[iii], *insignificant*[iv] and *unidentified source*[v].

Pharmacist's intervention

After the screening, pDDIs classified as *major* and *moderate* were assessed by a pharmacist, and for clinically relevant pDDIs recommendations in written form were prepared for the physicians. In addition to these recommendations, information leaflets according to *Pharmavista* on the possible ADR, the clinical management, the mechanism and literature references regarding the DDI were sent to the physicians. They were asked to give written feedback on the acceptance or rejection of the recommendation. In addition, within the second part of the study, physicians were asked to assess the clinical relevance of the pDDI themselves.

Implementation during hospitalization was verified according to the medication prescribed at hospital discharge, which was checked for changes according to the recommendations. Concerning the interventions at hospital discharge, general practitioners were asked for details about current medication to prove the efficacy of drug changes due to the recommendation one year after the intervention.

Statistical analysis

Descriptive data were expressed as means with corresponding 95% confidence intervals (CIs), as medians and ranges, or as proportions. Data were analyzed with R for Windows version 2.2.0 (R Development Core Team (2005), R Foundation for Statistical Computing, Vienna, Austria).

---

i *Major* interactions may be life-threatening, or intoxication or permanent damage may be induced. Normally, these drugs should not be administered together.

ii *Moderate* interactions frequently cause therapeutic difficulties, but the combinations may be administered if the patient is carefully monitored (laboratory parameters, for example quick value, or clinical symptoms).

iii *Minor* interactions may cause increased or reduced effects or interactions only concerning a certain subgroup (for example patients with renal or hepatic failure, slow acetylizers).

iv *Insignificant* interactions cause mainly no or unimportant effects and no special action is required.

v Within interactions classified as *unidentified source* no medical literature is available. Only isolated cases are cited or even postulated, and their clinical relevance is unclear.

## Results

Dropouts and patient characteristics

Between February and May 2005 (intervention during hospitalization), 539 patients were enrolled. Of these, 37 (7%) patients were excluded (31 patients died during hospitalization and six patients were excluded due to gaps in their medical history). The median time between hospital admission and the registration of the drugs prescribed during hospital stay was four days (mean 5.1 days, 95% CI 4.7 - 5.6 days).

Between June and October 2005 (intervention at hospital discharge), data concerning 826 patients were recorded at hospital discharge.

The characteristics of the patients included in the study are displayed in Table I.

Table I: Characteristics of the patients included in the study

| Characteristics | | Intervention during hospitalization (n = 502) | Intervention at hospital discharge (n = 792) |
|---|---|---|---|
| Age - yr | Mean | 68.4 | 66.5 |
| | 95% CI | 67.2 - 69.7 | 65.3 - 67.6 |
| | Median | 71 | 69 |
| | Range | 17 - 96 | 17 - 99 |
| Sex - no. (%) | Male | 231 (46) | 404 (51) |
| | Female | 271 (54) | 388 (49) |
| Length of hospital stay - days | Mean | 13.0 | 9.3 |
| | 95% CI | 12.1 - 13.9 | 8.6 - 9.9 |
| | Median | 10 | 7 |
| | Range | 1 - 91 | 1 - 72 |
| Number of diagnoses | Mean | 4.3 | 4.5 |
| | 95% CI | 4.1 - 4.5 | 4.3 - 4.6 |
| | Median | 4 | 4 |
| | Range | 1 - 16 | 1 - 15 |
| Main diagnoses (according to ICD-10) - no. (%) | Diseases of the circulatory system | 137 (27.3) | 221 (27.9) |
| | Diseases of the respiratory system | 78 (15.5) | 54 (6.8) |
| | Diseases of the digestive system | 52 (10.4) | 109 (13.8) |
| | Neoplasms | 42 (8.4) | 61 (7.7) |
| | Symptoms, signs and abnormal clinical and laboratory findings, not elsewhere classified | 36 (7.2) | 22 (2.8) |
| | Factors influencing health status and contact with health services | 14 (2.8) | 45 (5.7) |
| | Diseases of the nervous system | 25 (5.0) | 44 (5.6) |
| | Diseases of the musculo-skeletal system and connective tissue | 20 (4.0) | 42 (5.3) |
| | Others (< 5%) | 98 (19.5) | 194 (24.5) |

95% CI = 95% confidence interval, ICD-10 = international classification of diseases, 10$^{th}$ revision, n = number of patients, no. = number, yr = year

## Prescribed drugs and prevalence of *major* and *moderate* potential drug-drug interactions

The number of prescribed drugs (and drug pairs) per patient as well as the prevalence of *major* and *moderate* pDDIs are presented in Table II. During the intervention period during hospitalization, less patients (n = 502) were recorded than during the intervention period at hospital discharge (n = 792). Due to a higher median value of the drugs prescribed to inpatients than at discharge (11 vs 6) the total number of *major* and *moderate* pDDIs was higher during hospitalization (567 pDDIs) than at hospital discharge (392 pDDIs). The prevalence of *major* and *moderate* pDDIs in proportion to the number of drugs was 9.8% (1.13 of 11.5) during hospitalization and 8.0% (0.49 of 6.1) at discharge, respectively.

Table II: Number of drugs and drug pairs per patient and the prevalence of *major* and *moderate* potential drug-drug interactions (pDDIs)

|  |  | Intervention during hospitalization (n = 502) | Intervention at hospital discharge (n = 792) |
|---|---|---|---|
| Number of drugs, excluding drugs prescribed "as required" | Mean (95% CI) | 7.8 (7.5 - 8.1) | 5.7 (5.5 - 5.9) |
|  | Median (Range) | 7 (0 - 21) | 5 (0 - 18) |
| Number of drugs, prescribed "as required" | Mean (95% CI) | 3.7 (3.6 - 3.8) | 0.4 (0.3 - 0.4) |
|  | Median (Range) | 3 (0 - 12) | 0 (0 - 5) |
| Total number of drugs | Mean (95% CI) | 11.5 (11.1 - 11.9) | 6.1 (5.0 - 6.3) |
|  | Median (Range) | 11 (1 - 26) | 6 (0 - 18) |
| Number of drug pairs | Mean (95% CI) | 70.1 (65.3 - 74.9) | 20.8 (19.3 - 22.4) |
|  | Median (Range) | 55 (0 - 325) | 15 (0 - 153) |
| Number of patients with ≥ one *major* pDDI | no. (%) | 22 (4.4) | 6 (0.8) |
|  | 95% CI (%) | 2.6 - 6.2 | 0.15 - 1.36 |
| Number of patients with ≥ one *major* or *moderate* pDDI | no. (%) | 284 (56.6) | 243 (30.7) |
|  | 95% CI (%) | 52.2 - 61.0 | 27.5 - 33.9 |
| Number of *major* pDDIs per patient | Mean (95% CI) | 0.05 (0.03 - 0.08) | 0.01 (0.00 - 0.01) |
|  | Median (Range) | 0 (0 - 3) | 0 (0 - 1) |
| Number of *major* or *moderate* pDDIs per patient | Mean (95% CI) | 1.13 (0.98 - 1.27) | 0.49 (0.43 - 0.56) |
|  | Median (Range) | 1 (0 - 13) | 0 (0 - 7) |

95% CI = 95% confidence interval, n = number of patients, no. = number

## Pharmacist's intervention

As a result of the pharmacist's assessment, 419 pDDIs were judged as clinically relevant (74% of 567 *major* and *moderate* pDDIs) during the intervention period for inpatients. 349 recommendations (including information about the DDI) and in 70 cases simply *Pharmavista* general information leaflets were handed out to the physicians.

Regarding the intervention period at hospital discharge, 258 pDDIs were assessed as clinically relevant (66% of 392 *major* and *moderate* pDDIs), and therefore 247 recommendations (including information about the DDI) and in 11 cases simply *Pharmavista* information leaflets were provided to the physicians.

Table III shows a summary of the recommendations. 47 (11%) recommendations during hospitalization and 29 (11%) recommendations at hospital discharge required a drug withdrawal, a replacement or a prescription of another drug. During the hospitalization intervention period, 130 recommendations were provided in addition to further advice to the general practitioner (111) and/or the patient (25) about the DDI and the possible ADRs. At hospital discharge, physicians were asked to transfer each recommendation to the general practitioners, and 17 additional advices about possible ADRs due to the DDIs were given to the patients.

Table III: Type of pharmaceutical recommendation concerning intervention to avoid *major* and *moderate* potential drug-drug interactions (pDDIs)

| Pharmaceutical recommendation | Intervention during hospitalization (total number of interventions: 419) | Intervention at hospital discharge (total number of interventions: 258) |
|---|---|---|
| Withdrawal of a drug - no. (%) | 5 (1.2) | 5 (1.9) |
| Withdrawal of a drug prescribed "as required" - no. (%) | 13 (3.1) | 0 (0.0) |
| Replacement of a drug by another drug - no. (%) | 30 (7.2) | 24 (9.3) |
| Replacement of a drug by another drug or withdrawal of a drug - no. (%) | 4 (1.0) | 1 (0.4) |
| Replacement of a drug by another drug or withdrawal of a drug prescribed "as required" - no. (%) | 13 (3.1) | 0 (0.0) |
| Replacement of a drug by another drug or to pause a drug therapy - no. (%) | 4 (1.0) | 0 (0.0) |
| Prescription of an additional drug - no. (%) | 3 (0.7) | 0 (0.0) |
| Monitoring of the possible ADR - no. (%) | 24 (5.7) | 38 (14.7) |
| Monitoring of the renal function - no. (%) | 22 (5.3) | 12 (4.6) |
| Monitoring of the blood pressure - no. (%) | 17 (4.1) | 18 (7.0) |
| Change of the drug application time - no. (%) | 18 (4.5) | 35 (13.6) |
| Determination of the end of drug therapy - no. (%) | 6 (1.4) | 1 (0.4) |
| Monitoring of the INR value - no. (%) | 62 (14.8) | 42 (16.3) |
| Monitoring of the potassium serum level - no. (%) | 77 (18.4) | 39 (15.1) |
| Monitoring of the drug blood or serum level - no. (%) | 6 (1.4) | 15 (5.8) |
| Monitoring of the glucose blood level - no. (%) | 24 (5.7) | 6 (2.3) |
| Verification of the indication - no. (%) | 5 (1.2) | 4 (1.6) |
| Determination of the maximum dose - no. (%) | 10 (2.4) | 1 (0.4) |
| Information provided about the pDDI only - no. (%) | 70 (16.7) | 11 (4.3) |
| Others (< 1.0%) - no. (%) | 6 (1.0) | 6 (2.3) |

ADR = adverse drug reaction, INR = international normalized ratio, no. = number

In 218 (38% of 567) cases of pDDIs during hospitalization and in 145 (37% of 392) instances of pDDIs at hospital discharge, no specific recommendation was provided by the pharmacist. In 148 (68% of 218) pDDIs during hospitalization and in 63 (43% of 145) pDDIs at hospital discharge, the reason to ignore a recommendation was based on a different judgment of the clinical relevance of the DDI by the pharmacist. For example, the co-medication of insulin and cardioselective beta-blockers, $\beta_2$-sympathomimetics as inhalants and cardioselective beta-blockers, low molecular heparin and low dose aspirin or corticosteroids as inhalants and diuretics are all classified as *moderate* pDDIs by *Pharmavista*, but they were not assessed as clinically relevant by the pharmacist. Other reasons to ignore recommendations were due to individual patient variables (for example time-limited therapy, serum potassium level being too high or too low, prescription "as required"), or pDDI-management was already undertaken by the physicians.

Acceptance of the interventions and assessment of the clinical relevance of potential drug-drug interactions by physicians

80% (278 of 349) of the recommendations during the intervention period at hospitalization and 73% (180 of 247) of the recommendations during the intervention period at hospital discharge were accepted by the physicians. No feedback was obtained in 12% (42) and 13% (32), respectively. 8% (29) and 14% (35) of the recommendations, respectively, were not accepted.

During hospitalization three recommendations concerning *major* pDDIs were not accepted. All three concerned a non-cardioselective beta-blocker and $\beta_2$-sympathomimetic as a local inhalant anti-asthmatic drug.

At hospital discharge two recommendations concerning *major* pDDIs (a non-cardioselective beta-blocker combined with a $\beta_2$-sympathomimetic as a local inhalant anti-asthmatic drug and an $\alpha_2$-sympathomimetic drug combined with a beta-blocker) were not accepted.

Out of 258 *major* and *moderate* pDDIs at hospital discharge 209 (81%) were assessed as clinically relevant by physicians, 15 (6%) as not clinically relevant and in 34 (13%) pDDIs no feedback was obtained. Two *major* pDDIs (a non-cardioselective beta-blocker combined with a $\beta_2$-sympathomimetic as a local inhalant anti-asthmatic drug, and a potassium salt combined with a potassium-sparing diuretic) were assessed as clinically not relevant by the physician.

Verification of physicians' implementations

Verification of the implementation was only possible in cases where drug regimen changes (withdrawal, replacement of a drug or prescription of an additional drug) were recommended. In the first part of the study (intervention period during hospitalization) 85% (60 of 71 reviewed cases) of the recommendations were accepted (no feedback 4, rejection 7). 47 recommendations were implemented during hospitalization, which correspond to 66% of all recommendations and 78% of instances, which were accepted. The second verification (intervention period at hospital discharge) revealed that two patients were deceased within one year after discharge and one patient changed his general practitioner and could not be located. In 85% (11 of 13 reviewed instances, which were accepted) the drug changes due to the recommendation were still substantive and the pDDI was still successfully cancelled one year after hospital discharge.

Summary of the pharmacist's intervention and the physicians' acceptance

Figure I and II summarize the interventions and recommendations in *major* and *moderate* pDDIs by a pharmacist and the physicians' feedback about the acceptance of the recommendations I) during hospitalization and II) at hospital discharge. We can assume that in 50% (during hospitalization) and 46% (at hospital discharge), respectively, of all detected *major* and *moderate* pDDIs by *Pharmavista*, intervention was accepted by the physicians.

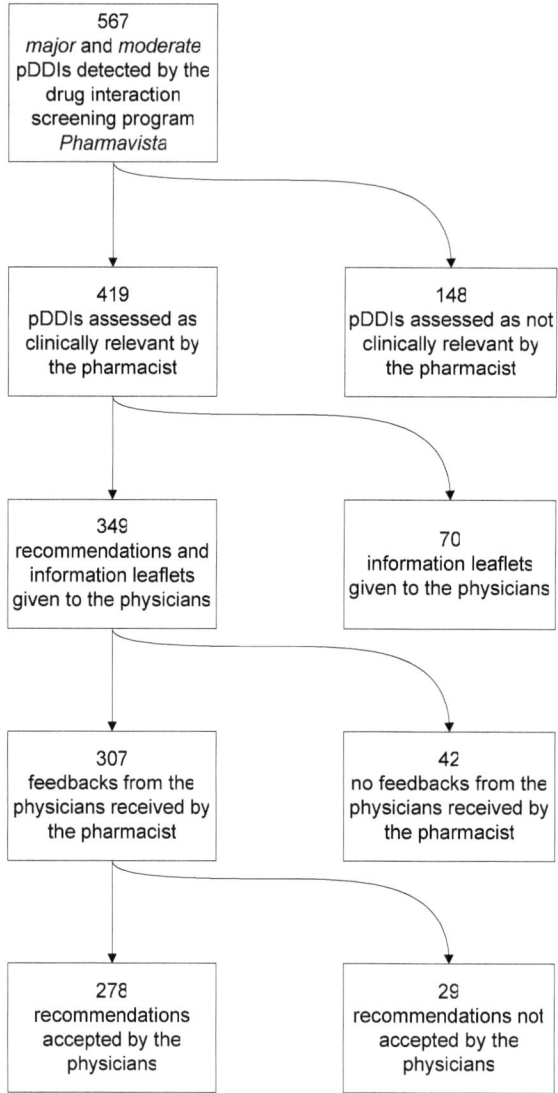

Figure I: Pharmaceutical interventions to avoid *major* and *moderate* potential drug-drug interactions (pDDIs) during hospitalization and physicians' acceptance of the recommendations

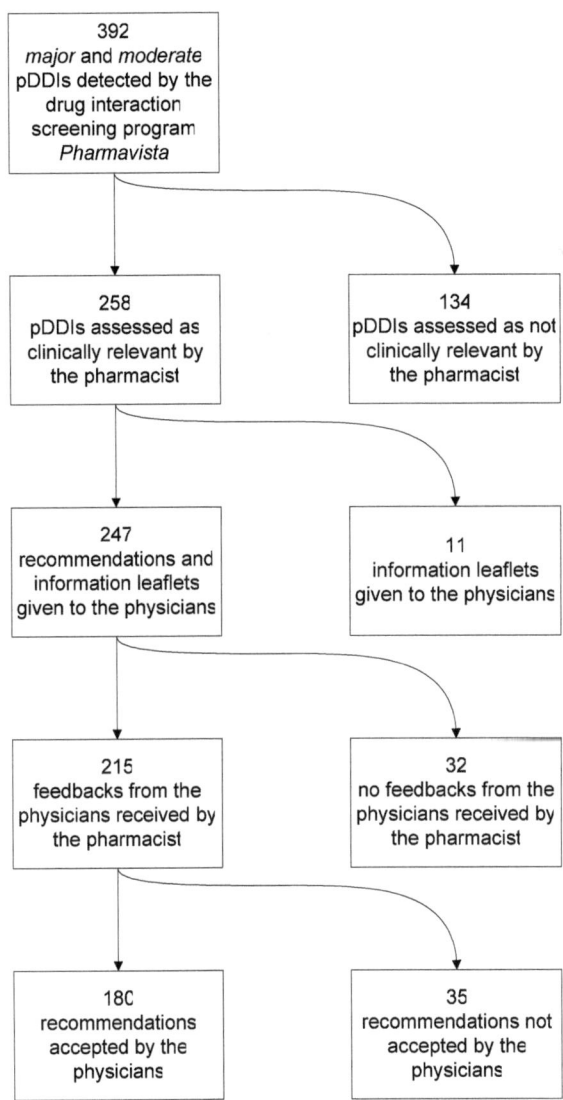

Figure II: Pharmaceutical interventions to avoid *major* and *moderate* potential drug-drug interactions (pDDIs) at hospital discharge and physicians' acceptance of the recommendations

## Discussion

Interventions made by pharmacists might reduce prescribing errors [19-21]. According to Leape et al. the presence of a pharmacist on rounds in a medical intensive care unit was associated with a substantially lower rate of ADEs caused by prescribing errors. The rate of preventable ordering ADEs decreased by 66% from 10.4 per 1'000 patient-days (95% CI 7 - 14) before the intervention to 3.5 (95% CI 1 - 5) (p < 0.001) after the intervention [20]. Direct association among clinical pharmacy services, pharmacist staffing, and medication errors was shown by an evaluation of almost half a million medication errors in 1'081 United States hospitals [21]. An analysis of the causes of preventable prescribing errors revealed that pharmacists should play a key role in the defences against prescribing errors, and that they should provide a supply role and monitor prescriptions to detect any errors that arise [22]. Clinical pharmacist involvement is desirable in the prescribing process together with CPOE systems with advanced clinical decision support, because CPOE systems can mitigate most but not all prescribing errors [23]. Potential DDIs should be predicted and dealt with by close teamwork between physician and pharmacist at the moment medication is prescribed [24]. Despite these recommendations and findings, a recent study suggests that the medication reviews performed by a clinical pharmacologist with special knowledge of DDIs and ADRs does not necessarily reduce drug-related morbidity or mortality [25].

The acceptance of the recommendations by physicians in the present study (80% during the intervention period at hospital and 73% during the intervention period at discharge) was comparable to 63% reported in an intervention study, in which written advice was provided. Acceptance in more than 90% of interventions was reported when direct spoken communication between physicians and pharmacists was possible [20, 26]. We assume that improvements regarding the acceptance of well-documented and easily manageable pDDIs would be possible. For example, three of 23 recommendations concerning interactions between statins and cytochrome P450 3A4 inhibiting drugs to replace the statin by a non-interacting statin or to pause the statin therapy during the anti-infectious therapy with clarithromycin were rejected by physicians. As reasons for these rejections they mentioned either absence of clinical relevance or rarity of clinical ADRs. To cite another example, three of eight recommendations concerning interactions between polyvalent cations and quinolone antibacterials to change the application time of the polyvalent cation were refused.

The clinical management of pDDIs mostly implies monitoring of either symptoms of a possible ADR or laboratory parameters. Only in 11%, a modification of the prescription was recommended. These findings concur with the results of an analysis of the nature and management of DDI alerts in Dutch community pharmacies, where 9% of all actions resulted in a modification of the prescription [27].

Drug interaction screening programs might be helpful tools to check prescriptions for DDIs. Although automated order checks offer possible benefits to patient care, the effect of such real-time warnings remains to be comprehensively assessed [28]. Previous research suggests that more warnings are ignored or overridden rather than followed [29, 30]. Diminishment of overrides was achieved by designating only critical to high-severity alerts [31]. About one third of all *moderate* pDDIs detected by *Pharmavista* were deemed to be not clinically relevant. This corresponds well with our evaluation study [18], which revealed a positive predictive value of 0.67 for *Pharmavista* using *Stockley's drug interactions* [32] as a gold standard. Other approaches to classify pDDIs not only according to the severity of a possible ADR might be more conducive to acceptance by physicians. An interesting assessment of DDIs was performed by a Netherlands working group [33] defining four core parameters: quality of evidence, clinical relevance, risk factors and incidence of the ADE. A management-orientated algorithm with four decision layers (severity, manageability, risk/benefit assessment and patient-related risk factors) was introduced and evaluated by another group [34]. Also the ORCA (OpeRational ClassificAtion) system takes into account the potential severity of the ADR due to a DDI, the factors known to increase or decrease the risk for an ADR and the existing management alternatives to avoid the DDI or to reduce the risk for an ADR by other means [35].

Hospitalized patients intervention can be provided at the point of prescription. In clinical practice DDI alert programs should be integrated into the CPOE system. Pharmacists should survey the overriding of alerts and interventions should be done, if overridden alerts are deemed clinically relevant [23, 26]. Drug prescription modifications shortly before hospital discharge are common. A pDDI check at discharge of the patients is substantial since the monitoring of patients after discharge becomes significantly restricted [10, 16].

### Limitations

Clinically manifest DDIs were not analyzed in this study and therefore we used the expression *potential* DDI. Data about negative clinical outcomes caused by DDIs are rare, but some retrospective studies have been published [36, 37] and showed increased risks for ADRs when drug prescriptions contain pDDIs. Intervention studies should be performed to investigate whether good clinical management of pDDIs can reduce drug-related morbidity or mortality.

### Conclusion

The management of clinically relevant pDDIs can be improved by physicians' advice of clinical pharmacists. Changes in medication due to pDDIs were found to persist up to one year after hospital discharge.

**References**

1. Einarson TR. Drug-related hospital admissions. Ann Pharmacother 1993 Jul-Aug; 27 (7-8): 832-40.
2. Bates DW, Cullen DJ, Laird N, et al. Incidence of adverse drug events and potential adverse drug events. Implications for prevention. ADE Prevention Study Group. Jama 1995 Jul 5; 274 (1): 29-34.
3. Classen DC, Pestotnik SL, Evans RS, et al. Adverse drug events in hospitalized patients. Excess length of stay, extra costs, and attributable mortality. Jama 1997 Jan 22-29; 277 (4): 301-6.
4. Lesar TS, Lomaestro BM, Pohl H. Medication-prescribing errors in a teaching hospital. A 9-year experience. Arch Intern Med 1997 Jul 28; 157 (14): 1569-76.
5. Lazarou J, Pomeranz BH, Corey PN. Incidence of adverse drug reactions in hospitalized patients: a meta-analysis of prospective studies. Jama 1998 Apr 15; 279 (15): 1200-5.
6. Fattinger K, Roos M, Vergeres P, et al. Epidemiology of drug exposure and adverse drug reactions in two swiss departments of internal medicine. Br J Clin Pharmacol 2000 Feb; 49 (2): 158-67.
7. van den Bemt PM, Egberts TC, de Jong-van den Berg LT, et al. Drug-related problems in hospitalised patients. Drug Saf 2000 Apr; 22 (4): 321-33.
8. Mjorndal T, Boman MD, Hagg S, et al. Adverse drug reactions as a cause for admissions to a department of internal medicine. Pharmacoepidemiol Drug Saf 2002 Jan-Feb; 11 (1): 65-72.
9. Pirmohamed M, James S, Meakin S, et al. Adverse drug reactions as cause of admission to hospital: prospective analysis of 18 820 patients. Bmj 2004 Jul 3; 329 (7456): 15-9.
10. Forster AJ, Murff HJ, Peterson JF, et al. Adverse drug events occurring following hospital discharge. J Gen Intern Med 2005 Apr; 20 (4): 317-23.
11. Krahenbuhl-Melcher A, Krahenbuhl S. [Hospital drug safety: medication errors and adverse drug reactions]. Schweiz Rundsch Med Prax 2005 Jun 15; 94 (24-25): 1031-8.

12. van der Hooft CS, Sturkenboom MC, van Grootheest K, et al. Adverse drug reaction-related hospitalisations: a nationwide study in The Netherlands. Drug Saf 2006; 29 (2): 161-8.
13. Jankel CA, Fitterman LK. Epidemiology of drug-drug interactions as a cause of hospital admissions. Drug Saf 1993 Jul; 9 (1): 51-9.
14. Smith L, McGowan L, Moss-Barclay C, et al. An investigation of hospital generated pharmaceutical care when patients are discharged home from hospital. Br J Clin Pharmacol 1997 Aug; 44 (2): 163-5.
15. Himmel W, Tabache M, Kochen MM. What happens to long-term medication when general practice patients are referred to hospital? Eur J Clin Pharmacol 1996; 50 (4): 253-7.
16. Cook RI, Render M, Woods DD. Gaps in the continuity of care and progress on patient safety. Bmj 2000 Mar 18; 320 (7237): 791-4.
17. e-mediat. Pharmavista - information for healthcare professionals. Version February 2005. e-mediat AG, Schönbühl, Switzerland; 2005.
18. Vonbach P, Dubied A, Krahenbuhl S, et al. Evaluation of drug interaction screening programs. Forum Med Suisse 2005; 8 S (Suppl 23): P15.
19. Hanlon JT, Weinberger M, Samsa GP, et al. A randomized, controlled trial of a clinical pharmacist intervention to improve inappropriate prescribing in elderly outpatients with polypharmacy. Am J Med 1996 Apr; 100 (4): 428-37.
20. Leape LL, Cullen DJ, Clapp MD, et al. Pharmacist participation on physician rounds and adverse drug events in the intensive care unit. Jama 1999 Jul 21; 282 (3): 267-70.
21. Bond CA, Raehl CL, Franke T. Clinical pharmacy services, hospital pharmacy staffing, and medication errors in United States hospitals. Pharmacotherapy 2002 Feb; 22 (2): 134-47.
22. Dean B, Schachter M, Vincent C, et al. Causes of prescribing errors in hospital inpatients: a prospective study. Lancet 2002 Apr 20; 359 (9315): 1373-8.
23. Bobb A, Gleason K, Husch M, et al. The epidemiology of prescribing errors: the potential impact of computerized prescriber order entry. Arch Intern Med 2004 Apr 12; 164 (7): 785-92.
24. Wiltink EH. Medication control in hospitals: a practical approach to the problem of drug-drug interactions. Pharm World Sci 1998 Aug; 20 (4): 173-7.

25. Mannheimer B, Ulfvarson J, Eklof S, et al. Drug-related problems and pharmacotherapeutic advisory intervention at a medicine clinic. Eur J Clin Pharmacol 2006 Dec; 62 (12): 1075-81.
26. Chan AL. Pharmacist intervention when interacting drugs are prescribed despite alerts. Am J Health Syst Pharm 2005 Sep 1; 62 (17): 1760, 1763.
27. Buurma H, De Smet PA, Egberts AC. Clinical risk management in Dutch community pharmacies: the case of drug-drug interactions. Drug Saf 2006; 29 (8): 723-32.
28. Kaushal R, Shojania KG, Bates DW. Effects of computerized physician order entry and clinical decision support systems on medication safety: a systematic review. Arch Intern Med 2003 Jun 23; 163 (12): 1409-16.
29. Payne TH, Nichol WP, Hoey P, et al. Characteristics and override rates of order checks in a practitioner order entry system. Proc AMIA Symp 2002: 602-6.
30. Weingart SN, Toth M, Sands DZ, et al. Physicians' decisions to override computerized drug alerts in primary care. Arch Intern Med 2003 Nov 24; 163 (21): 2625-31.
31. Shah NR, Seger AC, Seger DL, et al. Improving acceptance of computerized prescribing alerts in ambulatory care. J Am Med Inform Assoc 2006 Jan-Feb; 13 (1): 5-11.
32. Stockley II I, editor. Stockley's drug interactions. 6th ed. London, Chicago: The Pharmaceutical Press; 2002.
33. van Roon EN, Flikweert S, le Comte M, et al. Clinical relevance of drug-drug interactions: a structured assessment procedure. Drug Saf 2005; 28 (12): 1131-9.
34. Bergk V, Gasse C, Rothenbacher D, et al. Drug interactions in primary care: impact of a new algorithm on risk determination. Clin Pharmacol Ther 2004 Jul; 76 (1): 85-96.
35. Hansten PD, Horn JR, Hazlet TK. ORCA: OpeRational ClassificAtion of drug interactions. J Am Pharm Assoc (Wash) 2001 Mar-Apr; 41 (2): 161-5.
36. Ray WA, Murray KT, Meredith S, et al. Oral erythromycin and the risk of sudden death from cardiac causes. N Engl J Med 2004 Sep 9; 351 (11): 1089-96.

37. Juurlink DN, Mamdani M, Kopp A, et al. Drug-drug interactions among elderly patients hospitalized for drug toxicity. Jama 2003 Apr 2; 289 (13): 1652-8.

# Risk Factors for Gastrointestinal Bleeding: a Hospital-based Case-Control Study

Priska Vonbach[1], Rahel Reich[2], Friedrich Möll[1], Stephan Krähenbühl[3], Peter E Ballmer[4], Christoph R Meier[5]

1 Hospital Pharmacy, Cantonal Hospital of Winterthur, Switzerland

2 Department of Pharmaceutical Sciences, University of Basel, Switzerland

3 Clinical Pharmacology & Toxicology, University Hospital Basel, Switzerland

4 Department of Internal Medicine, Cantonal Hospital of Winterthur, Switzerland

5 Basel Pharmacoepidemiology Unit, Clinical Pharmacology & Toxicology, University Hospital Basel, Switzerland

**Abstract**

Introduction
Gastrointestinal (GI) bleeding is a frequent serious adverse drug reaction, potentially causing hospital admission and death. The aims of the present study were to investigate risk factors for a first-time GI bleeding leading to hospital admission and to assess the role of drug-drug interactions (DDIs) as a cause of GI bleeding.

Methods
We conducted a hospital-based case-control study at the Department of Internal Medicine at the Cantonal Hospital of Winterthur, Switzerland. 74 patients with a first-time GI bleeding in 2005 were matched to 148 controls on age, sex and calendar time. Data were analyzed by univariate and multivariate conditional logistic regression with calculation of the odds ratios (ORs) and 95% confidence intervals (CIs).

Results
Univariate analyses showed an increased risk for first-time GI bleeding in patients with international normal ratio (INR) values $\geq 4$ (OR 6.2, 95% CI 1.2 - 31.0), treatment with nonsteroidal antiinflammatory drugs (NSAIDs) (OR 7.0, 95% CI 2.8 - 17.2) and the combination of NSAIDs with glucocorticoids (OR 12.0, 95% CI 1.4 - 99.7). Anticoagulation alone in the therapeutic INR range was not associated with increased bleeding risk. Multivariate models including use of NSAIDs, oral anticoagulants, serotonin reuptake inhibitors (SSRIs) and/or proton pump inhibitors, body mass index, diabetes, hypertension and history of non-bleeding GI ulcer revealed a significant risk for GI bleeding for treatment with NSAIDs (OR 7.0, 95% CI 2.7 - 18.3) and with SSRIs in patients $\geq 70$ years (OR 9.0, 95% CI 1.1 - 75.0). Increased relative risks for GI bleeding were found in multivariate analyses for combined use of NSAIDs and glucocorticoids (OR 10.5, 95% CI 1.2 - 94.4) and for combined use of oral anticoagulants and NSAIDs (8 cases, 0 controls).

## Conclusion

The present findings suggest that a first-time GI bleeding is associated with INR values above the therapeutic range, but not with well-controlled oral anticoagulation in the absence of other risk factors such as DDIs. The combinations of glucocorticoids or oral anticoagulants with NSAIDs carry a high risk for GI bleeding and should therefore be performed only when the potential beneficial effects outweigh this risk.

## Introduction

Gastrointestinal (GI) bleeding is one of the most frequent serious adverse drug reaction (ADR) causing hospital admissions [1, 2]. According to Pirmohamed et al., drugs most commonly implicated in causing these admissions included diuretics (27.3%), aspirin (17.8%), nonsteroidal antiinflammatory drugs (NSAIDs) (11.8%) and warfarin (10.5%). GI bleeding was responsible for more than 50% of all ADRs leading to death [1]. Intake of anticoagulants is commonly recognized as a risk factor for bleeding complications. According to a nationwide study in The Netherlands the most frequent ADR-related diagnosis of hospital admissions was bleeding (8.6%), and the drugs most commonly associated with ADR-related hospitalizations were anticoagulants (17.8%) [2]. A Swiss study retrospectively analyzed all hospital admissions during one year and found that about 4% of them were directly related to ADRs. Analyzed by affected organ system, the most frequent ADRs were gastrointestinal complications (33%) caused by platelet aggregation inhibitors, NSAIDs, oral anticoagulants or digoxin. 21% of all ADRs were due to DDIs, whereof the combinations of NSAIDs and oral anticoagulants as well as the combination of platelet aggregation inhibitors and corticosteroids were most frequently observed [3]. Various former studies focused on the interaction between NSAIDs and oral anticoagulants as risk factor for GI bleeding. The short term risk for upper GI bleeding was six times higher (relative risk 5.8, 95% confidence interval (95% CI) 2.3 - 13.6) when anticoagulated patients were exposed to NSAIDs compared with the use of anticoagulants alone [4]. According to Battistella et al., 0.3% of the anticoagulated patients ($\geq$ 66 years) were hospitalized with upper GI bleeding per year, and the concomitant intake of NSAIDs was a risk factor for GI bleeding [5]. However, NSAIDs also seem to bear a risk for GI bleeding without concomitant anticoagulant therapy. An observational cohort study showed that the relative risk of upper GI bleeding for elderly users ($\geq$ 66 years) of non-selective NSAIDs was 4.0 (95% CI 2.3 - 8.5) [6].

The aim of the present hospital-based case-control study was to investigate risk factors for a first-time GI bleeding leading to hospitalization with a special emphasis on the role of drugs and DDIs.

## Methods

Study population and data source
The study has been reviewed and accepted by the local Ethics Committee.

This retrospective hospital-based case-control study was conducted at the Cantonal Hospital of Winterthur, Switzerland, a 500-bed teaching hospital providing primary and secondary care to a population of approximately 200'000 inhabitants. Between January and December 2005, patients admitted to the Department of Medicine were eligible to be included into the study.

Information on drugs prescribed at hospital admission (according to the anatomical therapeutical chemical (ATC) classification), demographic information (age and sex), admission date and length of hospital stay, main and additional diagnosis (according to the international classification of diseases, $10^{th}$ revision (ICD-10)), body mass index (BMI), nutrition risk score (NRS) according to Kondrup et al. [7] and laboratory parameters (international normalized ratio (INR) value and helicobacter pylori (H. pylori) test) were obtained from the electronic patient records.

Case definition and ascertainment
Cases were defined as patients older than 18 years, who were hospitalized due to GI bleeding as the main diagnosis. Patients with the following computer-recorded diagnoses (ICD-10) were selected: K25.0, K25.2, K25.4, K25.6, K26.6, K27.0, K27.2, K27.4, K27.6, K28.0, K28.4, K28.6, K92.0, K92.1 and K92.2. By reviewing the hospital discharge letters, individuals with a history of GI bleeding prior to the current hospitalization were excluded.

Controls
We identified at random two controls without current or previous GI bleeding per case, matched on age (± 1 year), sex and calendar time of hospital admission (± 1 month).

## Exposure definition

Patients were defined as current users of a drug of interest, when – according to the medical history – they were under treatment at hospital admission. Intake of oral anticoagulants (ATC B01AA) was taken into account at least until two days before hospital admission.

## Analysis of drug-drug interactions

Prescriptions at hospital admission were screened for DDIs potentially causing GI bleeding. As a result of our previous evaluation study of frequently used drug interaction screening programs [8], *Pharmavista* [9] was chosen to check prescriptions for DDIs. (The drug group of NSAIDs included both high- and low-dose aspirin). The program classified severities of DDIs into five categories: *major, moderate, minor, insignificant* or *unidentified source*. Major DDIs may be life-threatening, or intoxication or permanent damage may be induced. *Moderate* DDIs frequently cause therapeutic difficulties, but the combinations may be administered if the patient is carefully monitored. DDIs of all severities and the combination of *major* and *moderate* DDIs were included in the statistical analysis (see below).

## Statistical analysis

We conducted a matched analysis (conditional logistic regression model) using the software program SAS, version 8.02 (SAS Institute, Inc, Cary, NC). Relative risk estimates (odds ratios (ORs)) are presented with 95% CIs. P-values less than 0.05 were considered statistically significant.

For each case and control, the effects of the following potential risk factors for GI bleeding were assessed in univariate conditional logistic regression models: BMI ($< 25$, $25 - 29.9$, $\geq 30$ kg/m$^2$, or unknown), INR value ($< 2$, $2 - 3.9$, $\geq 4$, or unknown), NRS ($< 3$, $\geq 3$, or unknown), drug use such as oral anticoagulants (ATC B01AA), phenprocoumon (B01AA04), acenocoumarol (B01AA07), NSAIDs (M01A), cyclooxygenase inhibitors (M01AH), proton pump inhibitors (PPIs) (A02BC) and selective serotonin reuptake inhibitors (SSRIs) (N06AB); the diagnoses diabetes (ICD-10 E10 - E14), hypertension (I10 - I15), obesity (E65 - E68), disorders of lipoprotein metabolism (E78), metabolic syndrome and history of non-bleeding GI ulcer were assessed.

In a second step, we identified the DDIs of all severities and the DDIs classified as *major* or *moderate* in every patient and control, as well as specific DDIs between oral anticoagulants and SSRIs, NSAIDs, heparinoids, glucocorticoids, salicylates, tramadol or thrombocyte aggregation inhibitors, between heparinoids and salicylates, NSAIDs or glucocorticoids and between NSAIDs and thrombocyte aggregation inhibitors.

We then applied two multivariate models: a "pharmacologic model" including the drugs ingested by patients and controls, and a "DDI model" including the DDIs identified as specified above. Both models were adjusted for confounders defined as variables showing a significant risk for GI bleeding according to the univariate analyses. In addition, analyses stratified by sex, age (< 70 years, ≥ 70 years) and localisation of the GI bleeding (upper and lower) were conducted.

## Results

Characteristics of the patients and dropouts

During the study period from January to December 2005, the Cantonal Hospital of Winterthur registered 19'385 admissions, of which 24.3% (4'713) were allocated to the Department of Medicine, wherefrom 1.9% (90) due to GI bleeding as the main diagnosis. Sixteen cases were excluded (15 patients showed evidence for previous GI bleedings, one patient lacked sufficient clinical information). The detailed main diagnoses of the 74 cases are presented in Table I.

Table I: Main diagnosis of cases with first-time gastrointestinal bleeding (n = 74) according to the international classification of diseases, 10$^{th}$ revision (ICD-10)

| Main diagnosis | ICD-10 | Number of cases (n = 74) (%) |
|---|---|---|
| Gastric ulcer, acute with haemorrhage | K25.0 | 1 (1.4) |
| Gastric ulcer, chronic or unspecified with haemorrhage | K25.4 | 18 (24.3) |
| Gastric ulcer, chronic or unspecified with both haemorrhage and perforation | K25.6 | 2 (2.7) |
| Duodenal ulcer, acute with haemorrhage | K26.0 | 2 (2.7) |
| Duodenal ulcer, chronic or unspecified with haemorrhage | K26.4 | 16 (21.6) |
| Haematemesis | K92.0 | 8 (10.8) |
| Melaena | K92.1 | 9 (12.2) |
| Gastrointestinal haemorrhage, unspecified | K92.2 | 18 (24.3) |

n = number of patients

Further characteristics of the cases and of the matched controls are displayed in Table II. During hospitalization, 4 (5.4%) cases and 13 (8.8%) controls died (p-value 0.34).

Table II: Patient characteristics of cases with first-time gastrointestinal (GI) bleeding (n = 74) and controls (n = 148)

|  |  | Number of cases (n = 74) (%) | Number of controls (n = 148) (%) |
|---|---|---|---|
| Sex | female | 34 (45.9) | 68 (45.9) |
|  | male | 40 (54.1) | 80 (54.1) |
| Age | < 40 | 2 (2.7) | 4 (2.7) |
|  | 40 - 49 | 6 (8.1) | 12 (8.1) |
|  | 50 - 59 | 7 (9.5) | 13 (8.8) |
|  | 60 - 69 | 8 (10.8) | 17 (11.5) |
|  | ≥ 70 | 51 (68.9) | 102 (68.9) |
| Localisation of the GI bleeding | upper and lower | 2 (2.7) | 0 (0.0) |
|  | upper | 36 (48.6) | 0 (0.0) |
|  | lower | 35 (47.3) | 0 (0.0) |
|  | not available | 3 (4.1) | 0 (0.0) |
| Death during the hospitalization |  | 4 (5.4) | 13 (8.8) |

n = number of patients

Univariate conditional logistic regression

According to the univariate conditional logistic regression, we found a significantly increased risk for GI bleeding for various parameters: INR value ≥ 4 (OR 6.2, 95% CI 1.2 - 31.0), hypertension (OR 2.4, 95% CI 1.0 - 5.4), NSAIDs (OR 7.0, 95% CI 2.8 - 17.2), DDIs classified *major* or *moderate* (OR 3.3, 95% CI 1.5 - 7.2), pharmacodynamic DDIs (OR 2.0, 95% CI 1.0 - 4.0) and DDIs between NSAIDs and glucocorticoids (OR 12.0, 95% CI 1.4 - 99.7).

Furthermore, significant associations with GI bleeding were found for the following parameters in females: NSAIDs (OR 6.6, 95% CI 1.8 - 23.8), SSRIs (OR 6.0, 95% CI 1.2 - 29.7) and interactions between NSAIDs and glucocorticoids (OR 12.0, 95% CI 1.4 - 99.7). Males had a significantly increased risk for GI bleeding when they had hypertension (OR 3.4, 95% CI 1.3 - 9.4), took NSAIDs (OR 7.3, 95% CI 2.0 - 26.3), or drug combinations resulting in pharmacodynamic DDIs (OR 4.5, 95% CI 1.4 - 14.6).

We further stratified by bleeding localisation. The risk for upper GI bleeding was significantly higher in patients with diabetes (OR 3.0, 95% CI 1.1 - 8.3), and when they took NSAIDs (OR 8.3, 95% CI 1.8 - 38.7). Bleeding localised in the lower GI tract was significantly associated with an INR value ≥ 4 (OR 6.8, 95% CI 1.3 - 34.8), use of NSAIDs (OR 6.3, 95% CI 2.1 - 19.3), all DDIs (OR 2.9, 95% CI 1.2 - 7.1), DDIs classified *major* or *moderate* (OR 3.7, 95% CI 1.4 - 9.9), pharmacokinetic DDIs (OR 5.0, 95% CI 1.6 - 15.9) and pharmacodynamic DDIs (OR 2.8, 95% CI 1.2 - 7.0).

Patients ≥ 70 years showed a significantly increased risk for GI bleeding when they were exposed to NSAIDs (OR 6.6, 95% CI 2.5 - 18.0), to DDIs classified *major* or *moderate* (OR 4.1, 95% CI 1.6 - 10.9), to drug combinations resulting in pharmacodynamic DDIs (OR 2.4, 95% CI 1.1 - 5.5), and when they took NSAIDs together with glucocorticoids (OR 10.0, 95% CI 1.2 - 85.6).

## Multivariate conditional logistic regression

We applied a "pharmacologic model" (Table III) analysing the influence of various drugs (NSAIDs, oral anticoagulants and SSRIs as main parameters) on GI bleeding. Parameters were adjusted for the main parameters given above as well as for the use of PPIs, for BMI, diabetes, hypertension and for history of non-bleeding GI ulcer. Use of NSAIDs only showed a significantly increased risk for hospital admission due to GI bleeding (adjusted OR 7.0, 95% CI 2.7 - 18.3). Within stratified analyses, patients aged ≥ 70 years were at a significantly increased risk for GI bleeding when they received SSRIs (adjusted OR 9.0, 95% CI 1.1 - 75.0).

Table III: "Pharmacologic model"

|  | Number of cases (n = 74) (%) | Number of controls (n = 148) (%) | unadjusted OR (95% CI) | p-value | adjusted* OR (95% CI) | p-value |
|---|---|---|---|---|---|---|
| NSAID | 23 (31.1) | 9 (6.1) | 7.0 (2.8 - 17.2) | < 0.01 | 7.0 (2.7 - 18.3) | < 0.01 |
| Oral anticoagulant | 14 (18.9) | 24 (16.2) | 1.2 (0.6 - 2.5) | 0.61 | 0.7 (0.3 - 1.9) | 0.54 |
| SSRI | 6 (8.1) | 5 (3.4) | 2.4 (0.7 - 7.9) | 0.15 | 3.2 (0.9 - 11.4) | 0.08 |
| PPI | 18 (24.3) | 30 (20.3) | 1.3 (0.7 - 2.5) | 0.49 | 1.2 (0.5 - 2.7) | 0.66 |
| BMI (≥ 30) | 12 (16.2) | 22 (14.9) | 1.3 (0.6 - 2.2) | 0.57 | 0.3 (0.0 - 1.6) | 0.15 |
| Diabetes | 17 (23.0) | 25 (26.9) | 1.5 (0.7 - 3.2) | 0.26 | 1.5 (0.7 - 3.6) | 0.33 |
| Hypertension | 13 (17.6) | 12 (8.1) | 2.4 (1.0 - 5.4) | 0.04 | 2.1 (0.8 - 5.8) | 0.16 |
| History of non-bleeding GI ulcer | 8 (10.8) | 10 (6.8) | 1.7 (0.6 - 4.3) | 0.31 | 1.9 (0.6 - 6.1) | 0.26 |

*adjusted for NSAIDs, oral anticoagulants, SSRIs, PPIs, BMI, diabetes, hypertension and history of non-bleeding GI ulcer

BMI = body mass index, 95% CI = 95% confidence interval, GI = gastrointestinal, n = number of patients, NSAID = nonsteroidal antiinflammatory drug, OR = odds ratio, PPI = proton pump inhibitor, SSRI = selective serotonin reuptake inhibitor

The "DDI model" (Table IV) evaluated the risk for GI bleeding due to DDIs classified as *major* or *moderate*, pharmacodynamic DDIs, pharmacokinetic DDIs and the DDI between NSAIDs and glucocorticoids. Parameters were adjusted for BMI, diabetes, hypertension and history of non-bleeding GI ulcer. *Major* and *moderate* DDIs were associated with a significantly increased risk for GI bleeding (adjusted OR 2.8, 95% CI 1.2 - 6.4), and the combination of NSAIDs and glucocorticoids was also a significant risk factor (adjusted OR 10.5, 95% CI 1.2 - 94.4).

Table IV: "Drug-drug interaction model"

|  | Number of cases (n = 74) (%) | Number of controls (n = 148) (%) | unadjusted OR (95% CI) | p-value | adjusted* OR (95% CI) | p-value |
| --- | --- | --- | --- | --- | --- | --- |
| *Major* and *moderate* DDIs | 17 (23.0) | 11 (7.4) | 3.3 (1.5 - 7.2) | < 0.01 | 2.8 (1.2 - 6.4) | 0.01 |
| Pharmacodynamic DDIs | 18 (24.3) | 19 (12.8) | 2.0 (1.0 - 4.0) | 0.04 | 1.7 (0.8 - 3.5) | 0.14 |
| Pharmacokinetic DDIs | 11 (14.9) | 10 (6.8) | 2.3 (0.9 - 5.6) | 0.07 | 1.8 (0.7 - 4.6) | 0.26 |
| DDI between NSAIDs and glucocorticoids | 6 (8.1) | 1 (0.7) | 12.0 (1.4 - 99.7) | 0.02 | 10.5 (1.2 - 94.4) | 0.04 |

*adjusted for BMI, diabetes, hypertension and history of non-bleeding GI ulcer

BMI = body mass index, 95% CI = 95% confidence interval, DDI = drug-drug interaction, GI = gastrointestinal, n = number of patients, NSAID = nonsteroidal antiinflammatory drug, OR = odds ratio

## Discussion

Almost 2% of all admissions to the Department of Medicine at the Cantonal Hospital of Winterthur were due to GI bleeding. First-time GI bleeding was registered in slightly more male than female patients (54.1% vs 45.9%). The number of cases increased with age, more than two thirds of all patients admitted with first-time GI bleeding (68.9%) were at least 70 years old.

Our study suggests that the risk for GI bleeding under treatment with oral anticoagulants alone was not elevated (adjusted OR 0.7, 95% CI 0.3 - 1.9), if the INR did not exceed 4, and if patients were not exposed to other risk factors. However, if the INR value was ≥ 4, an increased risk for GI bleeding was observed (OR adjusted for BMI, diabetes, hypertension and history of non-bleeding GI ulcer: 5.6, 95% CI 1.0 - 30.3). This finding is in line with a recent Norwegian study reporting that 74% of patients treated with warfarin had – according to the authors – INR values above the therapeutic range at the time of GI bleeding [10]. According to a meta-analysis [11], the OR for major bleeds for INR 3 to 4 compared with INR 2 to 3 was 2.3 (95% CI 0.5 - 10.1), and did not reach statistical significance. However, the OR for INR > 4 compared with the INR 2 to 3 reference group was highly significant (OR 33.2, 95% CI 9.1 - 121.1). Various studies showed that the safety management and monitoring of an oral anticoagulant therapy is a difficult challenge for both patients and physicians. In such studies, the INR values were beyond the therapeutic range in 41 to 57% of the observation period [12-14].

Patients treated with NSAIDs showed a 7-fold risk (adjusted OR 7.0, 95% CI 2.7 - 18.3) for hospitalization due to GI bleeding compared to patients without NSAID treatment. The results of two recent cohort studies showed a 3.6- and 5.5-fold higher risk for current NSAID users of developing upper GI bleeding [15, 16]. According to another large case-control study the ORs ranged from 1.4 for aceclofenac to 24.7 for ketorolac, suggesting substantial differences between individual NSAIDs [17]. The annual incidence of NSAID-associated GI bleeding was also estimated in prospective outcome studies. Upper GI bleeding occurred in 3 to 4.5% of patients ingesting NSAIDs per year, and serious bleeding episodes due to bleeding of large blood vessel and/or gastric or intestinal perforation in approximately 1.5% [18].

In our study, patients treated with combined glucocorticoids and NSAIDs were exposed to an even 10-fold higher risk (adjusted OR 10.5, 95% CI 1.2 - 94.4) for GI bleeding. Similar results were published by Hallas et al. [15] (increase in risk from 5.5 for patients using NSAIDs alone to 10 for patients using NSAIDs and glucocorticoids), by Mellemkjaer et al. [16] (increase in risk from 3.6 to 7.4), by Piper et al. [19] (increase in risk from 1.1 to 4.4) and by Weil et al. [20] (increase in risk from 3.8 to 9.0). The combination of NSAIDs with oral anticoagulants is also associated with a higher risk of GI bleeding than use of NSAIDs alone. In the study of Mellemkjaer et al. [16], the risk for GI bleeding increased from 3.6 in NSAIDs users to 11.5 for the combination anticoagulants and NSAIDs. In a cohort study in NSAIDs users (≥ 65 years), the risk for hospitalization due to a bleeding ulcer was 12.7-fold (95% CI 6.3 - 25.7) for the combination anticoagulants and NSAIDs, and 4.0 (95% CI 3.4 - 4.8) for NSAIDs only [21]. In our study, eight patients were exposed to both NSAID and oral anticoagulants, but none in the control group, precluding the calculation of an OR. However, the OR for GI bleeding in patients treated with oral anticoagulants and NSAIDs compared to patients without these drugs is approximately 16.

Potential *major* or *moderate* DDIs resulting in increased risk for GI bleeding were significantly associated with a three-fold risk for hospitalization due to GI bleeding (adjusted OR 2.8, 95% CI 1.2 - 6.4). Gasse et al. conducted a nested case-control study to estimate the effect of concomitant use of potentially interacting drugs on the incidence of serious bleeding resulting in hospital admission or death. They calculated an adjusted OR of 3.4 (95% CI 1.4 - 8.5) in patients treated with warfarin and co-medication potentially increasing the effect of warfarin compared to warfarin alone [22].

The present results showed a significant association between age (≥ 70 years), treatment with SSRIs and hospitalization due to GI bleeding (adjusted OR 9.0, 95% CI 1.1 - 75.0). Published clinical evidence on the relationship between SSRI use and GI bleeding is limited to observational studies. Two retrospective cohort studies found no association between SSRIs and any recent bleeding events [23, 24]. In contrast, two other retrospective observational studies found a relative risk for hospital admission due to GI bleeding in SSRI users compared to non-users of 3.6 (95% CI 1.5 - 3.4) [25] and 3.0 (95% CI 2.1 - 4.4) [26], respectively. Van Walraven et al. analyzed three different groups of antidepressants that were classified as low, intermediate and high inhibition of serotonin reuptake. Their results showed a significant increase in upper GI bleeding with increasing inhibition of serotonin reuptake [27]. Moreover, available evidence suggests that concomitant use of SSRIs with NSAIDs or low-dose aspirin increases the risk for GI bleeding. In users of both medications, the risk markedly increased 12- to 15-fold and 5- to 7-fold as compared to nun-users of these drugs, respectively. The risk also increased 2.8-fold and 1.7-fold, respectively, when compared with SSRIs alone [28].

We also analyzed concurrent illnesses such as diabetes, hypertension, obesity, disorders of lipoprotein metabolism and history of non-bleeding GI ulcer as risk factors for GI bleeding. Unadjusted conditional regression analyses showed significant ORs for patients with hypertension (OR 2.4, 95% CI 1.0 - 5.5) or diabetes in male patients (OR 3.1, 95% CI 1.1 - 8.3). However, after adjusting for confounders, the statistical significance for both, hypertension (adjusted OR 2.1, 95% CI 0.8 - 5.8) and diabetes in male patients (adjusted OR 3.0, 95% CI 0.8 - 11.1) was lost due to a loss of power, but with very similar point estimates. The conclusion in a recent review supports these data, stating that hypertension may not be an independent risk factor for anticoagulant-related bleeding, when other risk factors were controlled for [29]. On the other hand, the presence of co-morbidities in patients with actual GI bleeding is associated with an increased mortality [30].

Limitations
Any epidemiologic studies may be subject to limitations such as confounding. Our data were retrieved from electronic medical records, and therefore some laboratory parameters such as INR values and H. pylori tests lacked especially for control patients. In addition, possible misclassification of diagnoses and incomplete patient records has to be considered. Recent studies showed discrepancies of up to 40 to 50% of patients' medication by comparing medical records and patient-reported use of drugs [31-33]. For non-prescription NSAIDs, disagreement was found even in 74% of patients' medication [33], and a systematic review found that up to 61% of patients had at least one omission error in prescription medication histories [34].

No statement about the GI bleeding risk for individual NSAIDs was possible in our study due to the small number of cases. A meta-analysis suggested that ibuprofen, followed by diclofenac bear the lowest risk for GI bleeding. Azapropazone, tolmetin, ketoprofen, and piroxicam ranked highest for risk where indometacin, naproxen, sulindac, and aspirin occupied intermediate positions [35]. According to a case-control study, ketorolac was associated with the highest risk followed by piroxicam, indometacin, ketoprofen and naproxen. Lower risks were found for aceclofenac, ibuprofen, nimesulide and diclofenac [17].

In our study, doses and durations of exposure to the drugs were not taken into consideration. In previous studies, increasing doses were shown to be a risk factor for upper GI bleeding [17] especially for ibuprofen and naproxen [16].

Finally, the number of cases (n = 74) and matched controls (n = 148) was rather small.

Conclusion

The results of this small hospital-based case-control analysis suggest that first-time GI bleeding is associated with high INR values, but not necessarily with oral anticoagulation alone if other risk factors such as DDIs are excluded. Although oral anticoagulants and NSAIDs as well as glucocorticoids and NSAIDs are frequently prescribed concomitantly in daily practice, our results emphasize the problems related to the combined use of these drugs. Strategies for reducing GI bleedings include better monitoring of INR values, careful dose adjustment and prescription of non-interacting drugs.

**References**

1. Pirmohamed M, James S, Meakin S, et al. Adverse drug reactions as cause of admission to hospital: prospective analysis of 18 820 patients. Bmj 2004 Jul 3; 329 (7456): 15-9.
2. van der Hooft CS, Sturkenboom MC, van Grootheest K, et al. Adverse drug reaction-related hospitalisations: a nationwide study in The Netherlands. Drug Saf 2006; 29 (2): 161-8.
3. Lepori V, Perren A, Marone C. [Adverse internal medicine drug effects at hospital admission]. Schweiz Med Wochenschr 1999 Jun 19; 129 (24): 915-22.
4. Knijff-Dutmer EA, Schut GA, van de Laar MA. Concomitant coumarin-NSAID therapy and risk for bleeding. Ann Pharmacother 2003 Jan; 37 (1): 12-6.
5. Battistella M, Mamdami MM, Juurlink DN, et al. Risk of upper gastrointestinal hemorrhage in warfarin users treated with nonselective NSAIDs or COX-2 inhibitors. Arch Intern Med 2005 Jan 24; 165 (2): 189-92.
6. Mamdani M, Rochon PA, Juurlink DN, et al. Observational study of upper gastrointestinal haemorrhage in elderly patients given selective cyclo-oxygenase-2 inhibitors or conventional non-steroidal anti-inflammatory drugs. Bmj 2002 Sep 21; 325 (7365): 624.
7. Kondrup J, Allison SP, Elia M, et al. ESPEN guidelines for nutrition screening 2002. Clin Nutr 2003 Aug; 22 (4): 415-21.
8. Vonbach P, Dubied A, Krahenbuhl S, et al. Evaluation of drug interaction screening programs. Forum Med Suisse 2005; 8 S (Suppl 23): P15.
9. e-mediat. Pharmavista - information for healthcare professionals. Version February 2005. e-mediat AG, Schönbühl, Switzerland; 2005.
10. Breen AB, Vaskinn TE, Reikvam A, et al. [Warfarin treatment and bleeding]. Tidsskr Nor Laegeforen 2003 Jun 26; 123 (13-14): 1835-7.
11. Reynolds MW, Fahrbach K, Hauch O, et al. Warfarin anticoagulation and outcomes in patients with atrial fibrillation: a systematic review and meta-analysis. Chest 2004 Dec; 126 (6): 1938-45.
12. Fihn SD, Gadisseur AA, Pasterkamp E, et al. Comparison of control and stability of oral anticoagulant therapy using acenocoumarol versus phenprocoumon. Thromb Haemost 2003 Aug; 90 (2): 260-6.

13. Mahe I, Bal Dit Sollier C, Duru G, et al. [Use and monitoring of vitamin K antagonists in everyday medical practice.]. Presse Med 2006 Dec; 35 (12 Pt 1): 1797-803.
14. Neree C. Quality of oral anticoagulation in patients with atrial fibrillation: A cross-sectional study in general practice. Eur J Gen Pract 2006; 12 (4): 163-8.
15. Hallas J, Lauritsen J, Villadsen HD, et al. Nonsteroidal anti-inflammatory drugs and upper gastrointestinal bleeding, identifying high-risk groups by excess risk estimates. Scand J Gastroenterol 1995 May; 30 (5): 438-44.
16. Mellemkjaer L, Blot WJ, Sorensen HT, et al. Upper gastrointestinal bleeding among users of NSAIDs: a population-based cohort study in Denmark. Br J Clin Pharmacol 2002 Feb; 53 (2): 173-81.
17. Laporte JR, Ibanez L, Vidal X, et al. Upper gastrointestinal bleeding associated with the use of NSAIDs: newer versus older agents. Drug Saf 2004; 27 (6): 411-20.
18. Laine L. Approaches to nonsteroidal anti-inflammatory drug use in the high-risk patient. Gastroenterology 2001 Feb; 120 (3): 594-606.
19. Piper JM, Ray WA, Daugherty JR, et al. Corticosteroid use and peptic ulcer disease: role of nonsteroidal anti-inflammatory drugs. Ann Intern Med 1991 May 1; 114 (9): 735-40.
20. Weil J, Langman MJ, Wainwright P, et al. Peptic ulcer bleeding: accessory risk factors and interactions with non-steroidal anti-inflammatory drugs. Gut 2000 Jan; 46 (1): 27-31.
21. Shorr RI, Ray WA, Daugherty JR, et al. Concurrent use of nonsteroidal anti-inflammatory drugs and oral anticoagulants places elderly persons at high risk for hemorrhagic peptic ulcer disease. Arch Intern Med 1993 Jul 26; 153 (14): 1665-70.
22. Gasse C, Hollowell J, Meier CR, et al. Drug interactions and risk of acute bleeding leading to hospitalisation or death in patients with chronic atrial fibrillation treated with warfarin. Thromb Haemost 2005 Sep; 94 (3): 537-43.
23. Dunn NR, Pearce GL, Shakir SA. Association between SSRIs and upper gastrointestinal bleeding. SSRIs are no more likely than other drugs to cause such bleeding. Bmj 2000 May 20; 320 (7246): 1405-6.

24. Layton D, Clark DW, Pearce GL, et al. Is there an association between selective serotonin reuptake inhibitors and risk of abnormal bleeding? Results from a cohort study based on prescription event monitoring in England. Eur J Clin Pharmacol 2001 May; 57 (2): 167-76.
25. Dalton SO, Johansen C, Mellemkjaer L, et al. Use of selective serotonin reuptake inhibitors and risk of upper gastrointestinal tract bleeding: a population-based cohort study. Arch Intern Med 2003 Jan 13; 163 (1): 59-64.
26. de Abajo FJ, Rodriguez LA, Montero D. Association between selective serotonin reuptake inhibitors and upper gastrointestinal bleeding: population based case-control study. Bmj 1999 Oct 23; 319 (7217): 1106-9.
27. van Walraven C, Mamdani MM, Wells PS, et al. Inhibition of serotonin reuptake by antidepressants and upper gastrointestinal bleeding in elderly patients: retrospective cohort study. Bmj 2001 Sep 22; 323 (7314): 655-8.
28. Yuan Y, Tsoi K, Hunt RH. Selective serotonin reuptake inhibitors and risk of upper GI bleeding: confusion or confounding? Am J Med 2006 Sep; 119 (9): 719-27.
29. Landefeld CS, Beyth RJ. Anticoagulant-related bleeding: clinical epidemiology, prediction, and prevention. Am J Med 1993 Sep; 95 (3): 315-28.
30. Rockall TA, Logan RF, Devlin HB, et al. Risk assessment after acute upper gastrointestinal haemorrhage. Gut 1996 Mar; 38 (3): 316-21.
31. Lau HS, Florax C, Porsius AJ, et al. The completeness of medication histories in hospital medical records of patients admitted to general internal medicine wards. Br J Clin Pharmacol 2000 Jun; 49 (6): 597-603.
32. Cornish PL, Knowles SR, Marchesano R, et al. Unintended medication discrepancies at the time of hospital admission. Arch Intern Med 2005 Feb 28; 165 (4): 424-9.
33. Abdolrasulnia M, Weichold N, Shewchuk R, et al. Agreement between medical record documentation and patient-reported use of nonsteroidal anti-inflammatory drugs. Am J Health Syst Pharm 2006 Apr 15; 63 (8): 744-7.
34. Tam VC, Knowles SR, Cornish PL, et al. Frequency, type and clinical importance of medication history errors at admission to hospital: a systematic review. Cmaj 2005 Aug 30; 173 (5): 510-5.

35. Henry D, Lim LL, Garcia Rodriguez LA, et al. Variability in risk of gastrointestinal complications with individual non-steroidal anti-inflammatory drugs: results of a collaborative meta-analysis. Bmj 1996 Jun 22; 312 (7046): 1563-6.

## 5 Conclusions

Our studies highlight the importance of potential drug-drug interactions (pDDIs) as a contributing factor in drug safety. Improvements regarding the awareness of pDDIs and a strict management should be implemented. Prescribing drugs with a low risk for pDDIs as well as careful monitoring for adverse drug reactions (ADRs) are important measures in the prevention of harm associated with pDDIs.

Drug interaction screening programs
Drug interaction screening programs are helpful tools to check prescriptions for pDDIs. Although automated order checks offer possible benefits to patient care, the effect of such real-time warnings remains to be comprehensively assessed [1]. In agreement with previous research [2, 3], the quality of these programs should be assessed before the implementation of a drug interaction screening program.

Our evaluation study of frequently used drug interaction screening programs showed that they vary not only in update frequencies, search and filter functions and severity classifications, but also regarding the quality of information provided within the interaction monographs and regarding the completeness and nomenclature of the drug list. Furthermore, sensitivity, specificity, positive and negative predictive value are of major importance. Pharmavista offers the most sophisticated information about DDI mechanism and clinical management, the highest sensitivity, a high negative predictive value and also an acceptable positive predictive value and can therefore be recommended. Our intervention study showed that one third of all *moderate* pDDIs detected by *Pharmavista* were deemed not to be clinically relevant. This corresponds well with the results of the evaluation study, which revealed a positive predictive value of 0.67 for *Pharmavista*.

Approaches not only including the severity classification of a possible ADR might be more acceptable by physicians. An interesting assessment of DDIs was performed by a Netherlands working group [4] defining four core parameters: quality of evidence, clinical relevance, risk factors and incidence of ADRs. A management-orientated algorithm with four decision layers (severity, manageability, risk/benefit assessment and patient-related risk factors) was introduced and evaluated by Bergk et al. [5]. Also the OpeRational ClassificAtion (ORCA) system takes into account the potential severity of the ADR due to a DDI, the factors known to increase or decrease the risk for an ADR and the existing management alternatives to avoid the DDI or to reduce the risk for an ADR by other means [6].

Prevalence of potential drug-drug interactions and pharmacist interventions

The main focus of this thesis was to elucidate the importance of clinically relevant pDDIs in the Medical Department of the Cantonal Hospital of Baden and to improve the clinical management of pDDIs by a pharmacist intervention during hospitalization and at hospital discharge. The analysis revealed that the quantity of prescribed drugs increased between hospital admission and patient discharge by 50%, but the number of *major* and *moderate* pDDIs per patient did not increase. In fact, the number of pDDI per drug pair administered was reduced by 50%. 47% of all *major* and *moderate* pDDIs at discharge were due to medication changes during hospitalization. Several deficiencies were detected regarding the management of clinically relevant pDDIs.

In the following section, the goal was the improvement of the clinical management of pDDIs by means of pharmacist intervention. For hospitalized patients, 74% of all detected *major* and *moderate* pDDIs by *Pharmavista* were judged as clinically relevant by the pharmacist. 80% of the recommendations were accepted and implemented by the physicians. During the intervention period at hospital discharge, 66% of all *major* and *moderate* pDDIs were assessed as clinically relevant by the pharmacist, and 73% of the recommendations were accepted by the physicians. One year after hospital discharge, 85% of the drug changes due to the recommendations were still persistent.

Overall, in 50% and 46%, respectively, of all *major* and *moderate* pDDIs detected by the drug interaction screening program *Pharmavista* a clinical management was provided by the physicians. It mostly implied a monitoring of either symptoms of a possible ADR or laboratory parameters. Only in 11 to 12% of the cases, a drug change was recommended.

We assume that the management of clinically relevant pDDIs can be improved by physicians' advice of clinical pharmacists. Changes in medication due to pDDIs are persistent even one year after hospital discharge. Clinical pharmacist involvement is desirable in the prescribing process together with computerized physician order entry (CPOE) systems with advanced clinical decision support, because CPOE systems can mitigate most but not all prescribing errors [12].

Potential drug-drug interactions as risk factors for gastrointestinal bleeding

The last part of this thesis focused on a serious – and potentially drug-related – complication. Gastrointestinal (GI) bleeding is one of the most frequent and serious ADRs causing hospital admissions [13, 14]. According to Pirmohamed et al., GI bleeding was responsible for more then 50% of all ADRs leading to death [13]. Our results suggest that first-time GI bleeding is associated with international normalized ratio (INR) values above the therapeutic range, but not with well-controlled oral anticoagulation in the absence of other risk factors such as DDIs. Increased relative risks for GI bleeding were found in multivariate analyses for combined use of NSAIDs and glucocorticoids and for combined use of oral anticoagulants and NSAIDs. Although oral anticoagulants and/or glucocorticoids are frequently prescribed concomitantly with NSAIDs, our results emphasize the hazard of these combinations and the need for rigid INR control.

References

1. Kaushal R, Shojania KG, Bates DW. Effects of computerized physician order entry and clinical decision support systems on medication safety: a systematic review. Arch Intern Med 2003 Jun 23; 163 (12): 1409-16.
2. Weingart SN, Toth M, Sands DZ, et al. Physicians' decisions to override computerized drug alerts in primary care. Arch Intern Med 2003 Nov 24; 163 (21): 2625-31.
3. Payne TH, Nichol WP, Hoey P, et al. Characteristics and override rates of order checks in a practitioner order entry system. Proc AMIA Symp 2002: 602-6.
4. van Roon EN, Flikweert S, le Comte M, et al. Clinical relevance of drug-drug interactions: a structured assessment procedure. Drug Saf 2005; 28 (12): 1131-9.
5. Bergk V, Gasse C, Rothenbacher D, et al. Drug interactions in primary care: impact of a new algorithm on risk determination. Clin Pharmacol Ther 2004 Jul; 76 (1): 85-96.
6. Hansten PD, Horn JR, Hazlet TK. ORCA: OpeRational ClassificAtion of drug interactions. J Am Pharm Assoc (Wash) 2001 Mar-Apr; 41 (2): 161-5.
7. Hanlon JT, Weinberger M, Samsa GP, et al. A randomized, controlled trial of a clinical pharmacist intervention to improve inappropriate prescribing in elderly outpatients with polypharmacy. Am J Med 1996 Apr; 100 (4): 428-37.
8. Leape LL, Cullen DJ, Clapp MD, et al. Pharmacist participation on physician rounds and adverse drug events in the intensive care unit. Jama 1999 Jul 21; 282 (3): 267-70.
9. Bond CA, Raehl CL, Franke T. Clinical pharmacy services, hospital pharmacy staffing, and medication errors in United States hospitals. Pharmacotherapy 2002 Feb; 22 (2): 134-47.
10. Lada P, Delgado G, Jr. Documentation of pharmacists' interventions in an emergency department and associated cost avoidance. Am J Health Syst Pharm 2007 Jan 1; 64 (1): 63-8.
11. Dean B, Schachter M, Vincent C, et al. Causes of prescribing errors in hospital inpatients: a prospective study. Lancet 2002 Apr 20; 359 (9315): 1373-8.

12. Bobb A, Gleason K, Husch M, et al. The epidemiology of prescribing errors: the potential impact of computerized prescriber order entry. Arch Intern Med 2004 Apr 12; 164 (7): 785-92.
13. Pirmohamed M, James S, Meakin S, et al. Adverse drug reactions as cause of admission to hospital: prospective analysis of 18 820 patients. Bmj 2004 Jul 3; 329 (7456): 15-9.
14. van der Hooft CS, Sturkenboom MC, van Grootheest K, et al. Adverse drug reaction-related hospitalisations: a nationwide study in The Netherlands. Drug Saf 2006; 29 (2): 161-8.
15. Laine L. Approaches to nonsteroidal anti-inflammatory drug use in the high-risk patient. Gastroenterology 2001 Feb; 120 (3): 594-606.

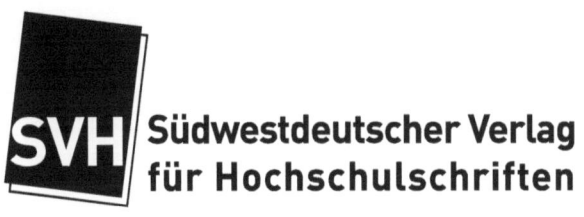

**SVH** Südwestdeutscher Verlag
für Hochschulschriften

# Wissenschaftlicher Buchverlag bietet
kostenfreie
## Publikation
von
## Dissertationen und Habilitationen

Sie verfügen über eine wissenschaftliche Abschlußarbeit zu aktuellen oder zeitlosen Fragestellungen, die hohen inhaltlichen und formalen Anspruchen genügt, und haben **Interesse an einer honorarvergüteten Publikation?**

Dann senden Sie bitte erste Informationen über Ihre Arbeit per Email an: info@svh-verlag.de.

Unser Außenlektorat meldet sich umgehend bei Ihnen.

Südwestdeutscher Verlag für Hochschulschriften
Aktiengesellschaft & Co. KG
Dudweiler Landstr. 99
D – 66123 Saarbrücken
www.svh-verlag.de

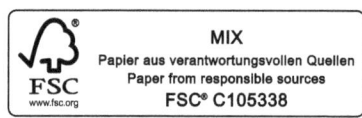

Printed by Books on Demand GmbH, Norderstedt / Germany